UNDER THE INFLUENCE OF MODERN MEDICINE

Terry A. Rondberg, D.C.

THE
CHIROPRACTIC
JOURNAL

UNDER THE INFLUENCE OF MODERN MEDICINE

Published by:
The Chiropractic Journal

Copyright © 1998 by Terry A. Rondberg, D.C.

Library of Congress Catalog Number: 97-078175
ISBN: 0-9647168-3-6

Printed in the United States of America
3 4 5 6 7 8 9 10 11 12

Table of Contents

**Dedicated
to the
Memory of Larry Webster, D.C.
1937 – 1997**

Dr. Larry Webster, known as the "Grandfather of
Chiropractic Pediatrics," established the
International Chiropractic Pediatric Association in
1975. He was a visionary who had real courage.
He was the driving force who laid the foundation
for chiropractic pediatrics credibility and clinical
training, which has improved the quality of life for
millions of children. He never compromised his
principles and was driven by his love for humanity.
His spirit will live on in the heart of every child
whose life he touched. Because of Larry, the world
is a healthier and better place to live in.

What the Readers are Saying

It is hard to refute the facts presented in Dr. Terry Rondberg's new book, *Under the Influence of Modern Medicine*. Chiropractors and patients alike will benefit greatly from the timely, documented information provided.

—*D.D. Humber, D.C.*
Senior Vice President for Clinics, Life University

Before you reach for your next pill, before you schedule another medical procedure, you must read Dr. Rondberg's latest book *Under the Influence of Modern Medicine*. This book proves that what you don't know can kill you!

—*Tony Palermo, D.C.*
President, Back to Basics

I feel a sense of personal relief now that this book has been written. In one volume the entire spectrum of medical deception is exposed in a credible articulate way. Only a Chiropractor could do justice to this subject and only Dr. Rondberg could do it with the passion and insight that he brings to everything he does.

—*Greg Stanley*
President, Whitehall Management Services, Inc.

I've read *Under the Influence of Modern Medicine* from cover to cover. All I can say is that if anyone still believed that medical science reigns supreme, they now must say, "the emperor wears no clothes." Thank you for writing a book that chiropractors can quote with authority and patients can use for educational purposes. You have done it again — given the world a gift of knowledge.

—*Veronica Gutierrez, D.C.*
Northwest Chiropractic Center

Dr. Rondberg's book is a summation of the dark side of medicine, the things that the medical lobby doesn't want the public to know; these are the failures and shortcomings of modern medicine. Dr. Rondberg has provided an excellent reference source for patients to understand what is really happening to them and their health.

—*Jeffrey A. Shay, D.C.*
Former Chairman, Medicare/Medicaid Committee, ICS

If you are looking for a book that will explain to your patients why we live in a drug-oriented world, why people turn to medication rather than natural remedies, you will want to read this book. The reader of this book will become enlightened and therefore more willing to support and refer to chiropractic.

—*David Singer, D.C.*
CEO, David Singer Enterprises

Under the Influence of Modern Medicine has picked up where *Confessions of a Medical Heretic,* by Robert Mendelsohn, M.D., left off. This is well referenced documentation of the hidden lies the medical profession has been feeding the public regarding drugs, surgeries, and so called "medical advances." A great expose of the orthodox medical scam that should be a must reading for all doctors and patients. Reading this book will reposition peoples' thinking from "treating illness" to "creating wellness."

—*Dennis P. Nikitow, D.C.*
Dr. Dennis P. Nikitow and Associates

This book is a well-documented exposition of some of the shortcomings of modern medical intervention as a basis for the preservation and enhancement of one's health. I hope that every medical patient will read this book as a thought-provoking exercise in informed medical consumerism.

—*David B. Koch, D.C.*
President, Sherman College of Straight Chiropractic

Dr. Rondberg's book *Under the Influence of Modern Medicine* is filled with factual evidence documenting the atrocities committed on people by the medical pharmaceutical industrial complex. It is must reading for anyone before they or a loved one visit another doctor or hospital if they want to avoid becoming one more medical casualty.

—*Matthew McCoy, D.C.*
Vice President, International Spinal health Institute

Dr. Rondberg provides a manifesto of sound evidence. An absolute must for any medicine cabinet.

—*Jay M. Holder, D.C. M.D., Ph.D.*
President, American College of Addictionology

In the 80's it was Dr. Mendelsohn's "The Medical Heretic," today we have a chiropractor who walk's the talk, and expresses what's really happening in medical care. You must read, absorb and shout the message that Dr. Rondberg delivers in his latest book *Under the Influence of Modern Medicine.*

—*Frank Sovinsky, D.C.*
Private Family Practice

In the shifting paradigm of modern medicine, this new information helps the reader to rethink and question traditional, and possibly harmful procedures. This book is truly a lifesaver. It is exceptionally researched and written and will change the way health care is practiced forever.

—*Theresa and Stuart Warner, D.C.s*
Post graduate faculty, Life University

Terry Rondberg's vital book, *Under the Influence of Modern Medicine* takes the medical bull by the horns. The medical myth has created more harm to our individual and global health, spirit, and culture than any other single story. Every patient must read this book. Every doctor and patient needs to read this book.

—*Donald Epstein, D.C.*
Developer of Network Spinal Analysis

Dr. Rondberg's new book will *finally* make the public aware of what *Under the Influence of Modern Medicine* really means in the cost of suffering to a trusting but submissive human race.

—*Harold G. McCoy, D.C.*
President, International Spinal Health Institute

Great... great... great. Every Chiropractor who lectures or talks Chiropractic daily with patients needs to buy this book ASAP in order to be loaded with statistical ammunition in the battle for the heart and soul of the health care consumer.

—*Guy F. Riekeman, D.C.*
Executive Director, Palmer Institute and Extraordinary Life Seminars

Foreword

Our society is experiencing a cultural crisis and chaos when it comes to health care — and trying to resolve it with a medical approach won't work. To paraphrase Einstein, you cannot resolve problems with the same level of thinking that existed when the problem was created.

We are faced with a major contradiction when we view medicine as "health care" because — in reality — it is *sick* care. When you take *sick* care and apply it to society as *health* care, you end up with a sick society. As a nation, we spend around one trillion dollars a year on what we call health care, yet our morbidity and mortality rates are unacceptable.

Many people (especially politicians) would like you to believe this health care crisis is fundamentally a financial one. But the high cost of health care is an effect, not a cause. Trying to control these expenses will merely redefine the problem — not correct it.

Correcting it will take a new level of thinking, or *paradigm,* in health care. There is no doubt a consumer-driven health-care revolution is taking place in the United States. People know radical change is needed, but have no clear vision of what that change should be.

Part of the problem stems from the fact that huge amounts of vital information have been hidden from the American public — information which is vital when trying to draw conclusions about proper health care for yourself and your family.

There is an important difference between knowledge and wisdom, and knowledge void of wisdom can be a very dangerous thing. Knowledge built the atom bomb ... wisdom will prevent us from blowing up the planet. The medical profession has accumulated vast amounts of knowledge over the years, but can lack wisdom in applying it.

Nature is incapable of programming for failure. We know the body is innately endowed with the ability to heal and regulate, and the nerve system is the master system and controller of that body. It stands to reason that if there is any interference with nerve function, there must necessarily be interference with the ability of the body to heal and regulate.

This wisdom goes a long way in determining what type of action, if any, should be taken when trying to achieve health and well being. So much of what is being pushed on us today in medicine interferes with the nerve system and disturbs the body's normal regulatory processes. This is NOT health care!

Amid the chaos, Dr. Terry A. Rondberg is a voice of reason and in this book, he raises that voice loud and clear. A true health care warrior, Dr. Rondberg has done a brilliant job documenting the horrible damage the current medical level of thinking has done to us. Much of the research in this book will have you shaking your head in disbelief. Believe it. Learn from it. Never let yourself or your loved ones be victimized because of ignorance of this information. Share it with others — their lives may depend on it. Join the revolution!

Patrick Gentempo, Jr., D.C.

Definitions

ADJUSTMENT: The specific application of forces used to facilitate the body's correction of nerve interference.

CHIROPRACTIC: A primary health care profession in which professional responsibility and authority are focused on the anatomy of the spine and immediate articulation, and the condition of nerve interference. It is also a practice which encompasses educating, advising about, and addressing nerve interference.

CHIROPRACTIC DIAGNOSIS: A comprehensive process of evaluation of the spinal column and its immediate articulations to determine the presence of nerve interference and other conditions that may contraindicate chiropractic procedures.

CHIROPRACTIC PRACTICE OBJECTIVE: The professional practice objective of chiropractic is to correct nerve interference in a safe, effective manner. The correction is not considered to be a specific cure for any particular symptom or disease. It is applicable to any patient who exhibits nerve interference regardless of the presence or absence of symptoms or disease.

HEALTH: A state of optimal physical, mental and social well-being; not merely the absence of disease or infirmity.

VERTEBRAL SUBLUXATION: A misalignment of one or more of the vertebrae in the spinal column, which causes alteration of nerve function and interference to the transmission of mental impulses, resulting in a lessening of the body's Innate ability to express its maximum health potential. Also referred to as nerve interference.

Chapter 1

The way to health

Everyone wants to be healthy. That's a "given" in our society. No reasonable person would prefer sickness, fatigue, and pain over a vigorous, vital and healthy body. But while the goal may be the same, people take different paths in an effort to reach it.

First, they can turn to the medical and pharmaceutical industries in hopes of finding health. They can visit medical doctors and surgeons, take prescriptions and over-the-counter drugs — all in an effort to treat their symptoms and diseases.

This path has created a multi-billion-dollar disease business in this country. But, according to almost every study done in the past few decades, it hasn't helped make us healthier. We're just as sick and out of shape as we've ever been. Major life-threatening diseases like cancer, heart disease, and diabetes are striking more people than ever. New epidemics like AIDS and Ebola are sweeping the globe. And so-called "medical science" isn't able to stem the tide.

In fact, the overuse, misuse and abuse of drugs and surgical procedures are adding to the death toll. Practices like chemotherapy and radiation therapy — labeled "barbaric" by many health practitioners — are, in many cases, killing the very people they're supposed to help.

Different path, same mindset

As people become aware of the failure of medicine to find answers to their health questions, they are looking for alternatives. They are turning to herbs and natural remedies to relieve symptoms and combat illnesses. By doing so, they are eliminating some of the dangerous side effects of the chemical compounds pushed by the pharmaceutical companies. Yet, although they have changed the type of pills they take, they haven't changed their way of thinking about health.

The old "take a pill and make it better" mentality is the biggest health problem we face in our society. We think that as long as we can take a pill that stops our nose from running, we're healthy; that if gulping down laxatives keeps us regular, we're improving the condition of our body.

But, if we are ever to achieve and maintain true health, we have to understand what health really is. We need to stop thinking in terms of treating illnesses, and start thinking in terms of creating wellness.

Most importantly, we have to realize that health is our body's natural state and the goal of health care should be to allow the body to function as it was designed to function. The body was created with all the mechanisms needed to maintain its health and — regardless of how much they want you to believe otherwise — medical doctors and drug company executives are NOT smarter than nature. They can hardly figure out how the body works, let alone figure out how to do it better.

Real health (not mere symptom suppression) is something we create from the inside, not something we can achieve from pills or surgical procedures. If we want to be healthy, our goal has to be to make sure the body can do the job it was meant to do, with as little interference as possible.

Is that a revolutionary idea? Not at all! It was around long before health care became big business. But healthy people don't ring up billions of dollars in drug store purchases and doctor visits, so the medical and pharmaceutical industries began promoting the idea that our number one health care goal was to treat diseases rather than increase our wellness.

Let's start with what health really means. After all, you can't work to achieve a goal if you don't really know what the goal is. A lot of people think health means not having a specific disease or symptom. If you don't happen to be in bed with the flu at the moment or be struggling with a bout of indigestion, does that mean you're healthy?

The most important thing to realize is that health is more than just the period between illnesses or the absence of symptoms. Health is judged by the way your body adapts to the physical and emotional changes in the environment.

For instance, if a healthy body is exposed to a flu bug, it should be able — if it's working right — to neutralize the effects of the virus. It'll also be able to adapt to the inevitable aging process without breaking down prematurely.

What happens when the normal functioning of the body breaks down and you get sick?

The medical approach is to prescribe antibiotics or pain remedies or other drugs to do the body's job for it. But those drugs do nothing to help the body regain its ability to do those jobs in the future. And, in fact, relying on pills to treat ailments can actually hinder the body's own abilities.

No drug or surgical procedure works to allow the body to do what it's supposed to do — and that's why they fail.

There are very few health care approaches specifically geared to helping the body achieve its own level of health. One of them, chiropractic, actually has that as its sole purpose.

Chiropractors aren't trying to eliminate symptoms and they definitely don't introduce anything foreign into the body. They work on the premise that the body's own inner wisdom is always trying to achieve a healthier state on its own.

The chiropractic philosophy is based on common sense. Even Albert Schweitzer, M.D., realized that, "Each patient carries his own doctor inside him. They come to us not knowing that truth. We are at our best when we give the doctor who resides within each patient a chance to work."

That's precisely what doctors of chiropractic do. They help give the "doctor within" each patient a chance to work by correcting vertebral subluxations which may be interfering with the natural flow of life energy over the spinal nerves to all the tissue cells and other parts of the body. When nerve interference is reduced, the body has a better chance of reaching its goal of better health.

So, the major health question we have to ask ourselves is NOT which pill to take, it's whether we want to create wellness or treat illness. If we continue to rely on medications we are merely trying to "take over" for the body.

Believe me, no pill on the planet can possibly match the power of the body to achieve health. Instead, work on getting your body truly healthy — through diet, exercise and chiropractic — and it'll do all the treating and curing that's possible.

Chapter 2

First, do no harm

One of the truisms of modern health care is that medical treatment can be hazardous to your health. In 1997, Lucian Leape, M.D. of the Harvard School of Public Health, reported that as many as three million people each year die or are seriously injured as a result of medical errors. That doesn't count the millions of people who are killed and injured by drug side effects and surgical complications which are considered the "normal risks" of medical procedures.

Reports like this, and others like it, rarely make it to the public. The billions of dollars pumped into the print and broadcast media by the drug and medical industries ensure silence about medical dangers.

Yet, the so-called "dangers" of non-medical health care fields gets frequent coverage in magazines and on television news shows. This has been particularly true of chiropractic, which champions a natural approach to health and is considered the number one "threat" to the medical monopoly in this country.

Rarely are medical failures mentioned by extremists like William Jarvis, Ph.D. and Stephen Barrett, M.D. of the National Council Against Health Fraud (NCAHF), which is widely considered the unofficial propaganda arm of the American Medical Association. After a federal court ruling that found the AMA and other medical organizations had conspired to disseminate misinformation about chiropractic in an attempt to destroy its "competition," the NCAHF became the front man for the attack.

Jarvis and his colleagues continually claim that chiropractic is dangerous and unscientific. Yet, the evidence they offer for their outrageous attacks appears to be a perversion of the truth at the expense of the uninformed health care consumer.

When the truth is revealed, an entirely different picture emerges. In fact, almost all medical and scientific research during the past several decades shows that chiropractic is extremely safe. However, chiropractic critics like Jarvis never refer to **these** reports. Rather, they put up a smoke screen of fear and lies to cloud the issue.

Thankfully, American health care consumers are becoming more sophisticated, demanding hard evidence for claims made by the medical profession. They know the medical community has an excellent record when it comes to emergency and trauma care. Stabilizing victims of accidents, heart attacks and other major health catastrophes is the rightful role of medical professionals and they carry it out as well as can be expected considering our limited understanding of the human body.

But when the medical and pharmaceutical industries try to expand from trauma care into "health" care — that is, the routine maintenance of health and wellness — problems arise.

Unfortunately, it's hard to convince some people they can live healthy, vigorous and long lives without constant assistance from the medical and pharmaceutical industries.

After all, we're all bombarded daily with the message "medication is good for you." Look around — newspaper and magazine ads, television and radio commercials, billboards, junk mail, product displays . . . even promotional brochures in food stores! The propaganda is everywhere and it's easy to associate those pills with the pictures of the happy, robust families which accompany the ads.

But, spend a few hours at a hospital and you'll get a truer picture. Children having convulsions because of reactions to vaccines. Women undergoing mastectomies because their doctors aren't informed of safer alternatives. Men undergoing triple bypass operations because their doctors never discussed healthy diets with them.

Then, look at the hospital parking areas reserved for the doctors and surgeons. BMWs, Lexus, Mercedes, Cadillacs. Obviously, there are those who are getting richer as America gets sicker.

We are "addicted" to the idea that medicine can bring health and it's a hard addiction to break. It's like smoking cigarettes for years, or drinking alcohol. At first, we refuse to believe we're addicted at all. The cigarettes or alcohol are our "friends." They're helping us, not hurting us. We close our eyes to the evidence that they are harmful and scoff at people who remind us of the facts.

The first step in breaking any addiction is to open our eyes, and our minds, to the possibility that we're wrong. We might do it reluctantly at first, with all the skepticism that comes with living in this modern age. But we try to put aside our pre-conceived notions and face the issue objectively.

That's the way everybody should approach health. If we aren't yet convinced we have the power within us to create our own health — if we still have faith that medical doctors and pharmaceutical companies are an essential part of healthy living — we need only agree to look at the evidence and judge it dispassionately.

This book presents some of that evidence. Each article is fully documented and contains information taken directly from dozens of medical and scientific journals. The articles clearly demonstrate the deficiencies and dangers of modern medicine, and the entire "disease paradigm" to help people achieve any kind of health for themselves or their children. But, since it pre sents stark proof that modern medicine has, in many instances, posed the greatest danger to health, these stories were often ignored by the mainstream press or suppressed by the drug industry.

The knowledge you gain from this book will open your eyes and give you the knowledge you need to make the choices which are best for you. If you have been trying to reach a state of health by treating symptoms and diseases, by rushing to medical doctors, by downing prescription or over-the-counter drugs, you'll see how vital it is for you to retrace your path and start again. It will show you why medicine should always be the last resort, not the first thing you turn to. It will give you strong reasons for practicing a lifetime wellness program with proper diet, exercise, chiropractic and other safe and life-enhancing health strategies.

> *"The fact remains, and the evidence proves, that 'bad medicine' hurts, cripples and kills more people in 24 hours than the chiropractic profession has been accused of harming in more than 100 years."*
>
> *— Terry A. Rondberg, D.C.*

Chapter 3

Cancer

N o disease is as feared as cancer. It one of the major causes of death in this country and, possibly even worse, it is associated with tremendous pain, debilitation, and despair. It strikes children and senior citizens, men and women, rich and poor . . . every age, race, economic class. No one, apparently, is safe.

This fear has sparked a billion-dollar cancer industry, with drugs, clinics, hospitals and research projects all making piles of money and empty promises. Yet, the only progress made so far on cancer has been as a result of anti-smoking campaigns. No drugs or therapy have helped reduce the overall incidence of cancer and many are now being shown to cause more problems than they could ever have solved in the first place.

Doctors admit defeat in war on cancer

In a report published in the *New England Journal of Medicine,* researchers admitted that, "Despite decades of basic and clinical research and trials of promising new therapies, cancer remains a major cause of morbidity and mortality... The effect of new treatments for cancer on mortality has been largely disappointing."

The researchers examined statistics on cancer death rates in the United States from 1970 through 1994 and found that age-adjusted mortality due to cancer in 1994 was six percent higher than the rate in 1970.

Yet, during this period of failure, the cancer industry has *grown* into a multibillion dollar business, with dozen of cancer organizations, research programs, and publicity campaigns being funded by both private funds and tax revenues.

The authors concluded that, "The most promising approach to the control of cancer is a national commitment to prevention, with a concomitant rebalancing of the focus and funding of research."

According to statistics compiled from the National Cancer Institute, American Cancer Society, and the Centers for Disease Control, cancer remains the second leading cause of death in the United States, behind heart disease. Today — 25 years and billions of dollars after the "war" began — 40% of people with cancer live at least five years after diagnosis — up a mere seven percent from the survival rate in the 1960s.

According to the American Society of Clinical Oncology, it is estimated that nearly 1.4 million new cancer cases will be diagnosed in 1997 and approximately 560,000 people will die from the disease.

These figures make it clear that the American people are not benefitting from the billions of dollars already expended for "research." If the answers have not been uncovered following traditional methods, it seems reasonable to fund alternative programs in search of solutions.

Time alone will tell who speaks louder: cancer patients and their families who are generally open to new possibilities, or large research institutions and pharmaceutical and medical companies that have little to gain and much to lose should cures or successful treatments be discovered outside their respective arenas.

SOURCES: Paper by the American Society of Clinical Oncology, presented at the Annual Meeting, May 17-20, 1997 in Denver.

"Cancer Undefeated," by John C. Bailar III and Heather L. Gornik. *New England Journal of Medicine,* May 29, 1997.

Americans spend big bucks but cancer care still poor

America spends more money on health care than any nation in the world, yet its citizens don't have the best health care. That's the conclusion of researchers from the U.S. General Accounting Office (GAO) who say that the U.S. tops the list in terms of per capita spending and the proportion of gross domestic product devoted to health.

Clearly, however, Americans aren't getting their money's worth.

"Many U.S. citizens assume that greater resources will lead to better care," the GAO researchers noted. "Yet the growing literature on comparative health care outcomes suggests that the high level of health care spending in the United States has not led to clearly superior results for U.S. patients."

The GAO study was published in the *American Journal of Public Health.*

Despite the fact that Americans spend more, the rate of survival for colon cancer, lung cancer, and Hodgkin's disease were similar in both the U.S. and Canada. In fact, the survival rate for lung cancer was slightly better for Canadians at the end of the 13-year study period.

The researchers concluded, that when it comes to these three types of cancer, "one health system is not categorically better than the other with respect to cancer outcomes."

SOURCE: American Journal of Public Health, August 4, 1997.

Chemotherapy actually causes cancer, studies find

According to scientific studies published in the *Journal of the National Cancer Institute,* chemotherapy may actually cause more cancer than it supposedly cures.

In the latest study, it was shown that patients who were subjected to chemotherapy were 14 times more likely to develop leukemia than patients who had not undergone the controversial treatment.

Cases involving more than 10,000 patients with Hodgkin's disease — dating from 1940 through 1987 — were reviewed for the research project. Although the treatment was successful in treating some cases of Hodgkin's disease, it significantly increased the risk of leukemia. Chemotherapy was also associated with a six times greater risk of developing cancer of the bones, joints, and soft tissue.

SOURCES: *Journal of the National Cancer Institute,* Vol. 87, No. 10, May 17, 1995, pp. 732-41. "Incidence of second cancers in patients treated for Hodgkin's disease," by Boivin, Jean-Francois, et al.

Journal of the National Cancer Institute, Vol. 87, No. 10, May 17, 1995, pp. 705-06. " "Body wars: effect of friendly fire (cancer therapy)," by Boice, John D. and Travis, Lois B.

Journal of the National Cancer Institute, Oct. 5, 1994 v86 n19 p1450(8). "Incidence of second cancers in patients treated for Hodgkin's disease," by Travis, Lois B.

Body may hold cancer cure key

For years, the medical and pharmaceutical companies have searched in labs to find a "cure" for cancer, yet we're still no closer to a solution today. It had long been rumored that the cancer "industry" wasn't unhappy about this as long as its current system guaranteed profits — BIG profits.

Now, however, several researchers have begun looking in the right place: the human body itself.

A study published in the *Journal of The National Cancer Institute* by researchers at the University of Maryland Cancer Center found that inter-leukin-10, a naturally occurring compound found in the immune system, may have potential as a treatment for cancers that have spread.

The researchers say that interleukin-10 seems to have little toxicity. The study shows, for the first time, that the compound seems to be effective in fighting cancers that have spread from their original site to other parts of the body. The researchers say it deserves consideration as a potential treatment for human cancer. However, they add that more studies need to be conducted.

The likelihood that additional studies will actually be undertaken is doubtful. Many scientists and health care advocates agree that pharmaceutical companies, research centers, and other profit-making medical concerns have a strong motive for stopping such efforts.

As health advocate and book author Jim Devlin noted in 1981, "Medical research will never find a cure for cancer. In fact, if it could find one, it might do everything in its power to bury it at the bottom of the deepest ocean. Why? Because cancer is big business, perhaps our biggest single industry."

As though predicting the work of the researchers, Devlin added, "No doctor cures anything. No hospital heals. No medicine truly makes one well. It is the force within one's own body, the life in the blood stream which effects all cures."

The information about interleukin-10 should have made front page news across the country, but instead, the public learned only of new drugs and surgical techniques to "cure" cancer. It will not be surprising, then, to too many people if research on the body's ability to cure cancer is not pursued — or if the findings discovered so far are suppressed.

SOURCES:"Compound in body's immune system may have potential to treat cancer," News Release, Maryland Medical Center, May 1996.

"Antimetastatic and antitumor activities of interleukin 10 in a murine model of breast cancer." *Journal of the National Cancer Institute,* April 17, 1996 v88 n8 p536(6).

"Bee Pollen and the New You," by Jim Devlin. 1981.

Doctors ignore simple way to prevent cancer

Despite continued evidence that people can greatly reduce their risk of cancer by eating properly, medical doctors often ignore the topic of nutrition when talking with patients.

Although numerous "cancer fighting" drugs are being introduced into the marketplace each year, the best "medicine" might be in the produce aisle.

That was the conclusion of researchers who published their findings in the *British Medical Journal.*

Technically described as a "Randomised controlled trial of effect of fruit and vegetable consumption on plasma concentrations of lipids and antioxidants," the research paper's conclusion was easy to understand. Basically, people who eat small quantities of fruits and vegetables can help protect themselves against cancer by increasing their consumption.

The study's authors asked 87 people who normally ate three or fewer servings of fruits and vegetables to eat eight servings over a period of eight weeks. Results showed that their blood concentrations of vitamin C and beta-carotene increased in direct proportion to the increased dietary intake of fruits and vegetables.

Concentrations of antioxidants at this level, said the authors, are likely to reduce the risk of cancer.

Yet, medical doctors rarely discuss diet with their patients, and few seem willing to recommend a good diet rather than write a prescription. This is partly due to a lack of education on the topic. Because the M.D.'s focus is on how to treat specific diseases with surgery or the more than 6,000 drugs now on the market, medical students are given virtually no training in nutrition.

SOURCE: British Medical Journal, June 21, 1997.

Researchers show selenium may prevent cancers

In 1988, the *Journal of the American Medical Association (JAMA)* published the **preliminary** results from a controlled experiment of high-risk men. The study found that the men who took aspirin had half the number of heart attacks as those in the group who didn't take it.

The study also found that those taking the aspirin suffered more strokes.

Days later, aspirin manufacturers — who make billions of dollars on a variety of over-the- counter aspirin products — saturated the airwaves with commercials claiming their pills prevented heart attacks. Within months, medical doctors around the nation were telling perfectly healthy patients to take an aspirin a day as a preventive measure, despite numerous reports which clearly demonstrated the potentially dangerous side effects of even low doses of aspirin.

In Dec. 1996, *JAMA* published a report from researchers at the Arizona Cancer Center, College of Medicine, University of Arizona. The study — which lasted more than six years — found that the participants taking selenium supplements had a 37% reduction in cancer incidence and a 50% reduction in cancer mortality.

Of the nearly 200 cases of cancer diagnosed, the selenium group had 63% fewer prostate cancers, 58% fewer colorectal cancers and 46% fewer lung cancers than the placebo group. There was not a single case of selenium toxicity reported in any of the patients being studied.

Yet, the medical community immediately issued dire "warnings," urging patients **not** to take the all-natural nutritional supplement!

In the same issue, *JAMA* ran an editorial by Graham A. Colditz, M.B.B.S., Dr. P.H., of Brigham and Women's Hospital and Harvard Medical School. In it, he stated, "For now it is premature to change individual behavior, to market specific selenium supplements, or to modify public health recommendations based on the results of this one randomized trial."

Information in the study revealed an even more startling fact: selenium was first associated with cancer risk in the late 1960s. Yet the billion-dollar "cancer industry" has never publicized that information and has never recommended supplemental selenium.

None of the major pharmaceutical companies markets selenium, which is normally found in health food stores for less than $7.00 per 100 tablets.

SOURCES:*The Journal of the American Medical Association,* December 24, 1996, and June 3, 1988.

Media advisory, Arizona Cancer Center, December 24, 1996.

Anti-cancer drugs linked to birth defects

Men and boys who are subjected to chemotherapy for Hodgkin's disease may end up with mutations in their sperm cells that could lead to birth defects in their children.

"This particular study is essentially the first clean demonstration that exposure of young men to certain drugs increases the frequency of sperm that are aneuploid," says biophysicist Dr. Andrew Wyrobek of the Lawrence Livermore National Laboratory in Livermore, California.

Wyrobek's research report, which was published in *Nature Genetics,* confirmed that the drugs can cause a deviation from the normal number of chromosomes in their sperm cells, called an aneuploidy. Aneuploidy is the cause for both a significant proportion of pregnancy loss and for chromosomal abnormality syndrome detected at birth.

According to the authors, an estimated four of every 1,000 live births are affected by aneuploidy.

The researchers evaluated eight men (ages 27 to 39) with Hodgkin's disease who were starting a chemotherapy regimen.

"The main reason we chose Hodgkin's disease was that it involves young men, and the cure rate these days is pretty high," says Wyrobek. "So we're talking about young men that are cured of their cancer and still may be interested in having children."

The men who had been subjected to the treatment had a 500% increase in the number of sperm with aneuploidy. Although the percentage of mutated sperm returned to normal levels several months after the treatment was stopped, the researchers remained concerned about the long-term effects.

They noted, "Each year more than 20,000 children and young persons of reproductive age are exposed to known mutagens in the form of chemo- and/or radiotherapy for cancer in the States.... there is growing concern that genetic defects are introduced in the germ cells of these young patients."

SOURCE: "Chemotherapy induces transient sex chromosomal and autosomal aneuploidy in human sperm," by Wendie A. Robbins, Andrew J. Wyrobek, et.al. *Nature Genetics,* May 1997.

Chapter 4

The plight of the elderly

One of the most vulnerable segments of our population is the elderly. Modern medicine has created the attitude that growing old is a disease which, in itself, needs to be treated. Many older Americans are taking up to 15 different prescriptions at the same time, and often their doctors aren't even aware of the potentially dangerous effects of drug combining.

Part of this is because doctors and hospitals will often recommend visits, drugs and tests simply because Medicare or Medicaid will pay for them. Recommending a diet and exercise program which has been proven to reduce the problems associated with arthritis doesn't generate income. Instead, the patient would merely get well and stop having to put in insurance claims for office visits and prescriptions.

The only way to perpetuate the profit-oriented medical industry is to make sure these people have to continue going to their doctors and filling their prescriptions. And the only way to guarantee that is to make sure they never are truly healthy.

Elderly exposed to too many tests

The use of diagnostic testing on Medicare patients increased by as much as 300% over a seven-year period, leading to a subsequent rise in medical treatments, according to an article in *The Journal of the American Medical Association (JAMA)*.

Diana Verrilli, M.S., of the Urban Institute in Washington, D.C., and H. Gilbert Welch, M.D., M.P.H., of the Veterans Affairs Medical Center, White River, Vt., and Dartmouth Medical School, Hanover, N.H., studied Medicare data to obtain information on all physician claims submitted from 1987 through 1993. These data represent physician services received by approximately 30 million elderly Americans in each of seven years.

The authors stated, "... The annual rate of diagnostic testing has increased rapidly for elderly Americans. The slowest increase was observed for abdominal ultrasound, approximately a 40 percent increase over seven years. The most rapid increase was observed for prostate biopsy, which occurred three times as frequently in 1993 as in 1987 ... The rate of diagnostic testing increased in every year (1987 through 1992) until 1993, when it declined slightly."

The researchers warned that there is a potential danger to over-diagnosing.

"Just as physicians have begun to recognize that more therapy may be harmful, physicians should also recognize that more diagnosis may be harmful," they wrote.

One of the most obvious dangers is the transformation of a person into a patient. "Although the risks of the tests themselves may be relatively small, the cascade of subsequent events may quickly spiral out of control, exposing patients to significant risks," the study noted.

SOURCE: "Diagnostic medical tests on elderly on the rise," Media Advisory, American Medical Association, April 16, 1996.

Researchers question need for annual flu shots for seniors

A scientific study by Israeli researchers has suggested that people over 65 years of age may not benefit from annual flu shots. The results of their study were presented at the annual meeting of the American Geriatrics Society held in Atlanta, May 7-11, 1997.

According to Haim Dannenberg of the Hadassah University Hospital in Jerusalem, the study revealed that subjects who had been given repeated flu shots had **lower** antibody levels than those who had not been vaccinated. The average age of participants was 72.

When the study began, the subjects — who had been vaccinated one year prior to the study — were tested for antibodies against three major strains of flu (A/Johannesburg, A/Texas, and B/Harbin). All showed levels higher than subjects who had not been tested.

After they received another vaccination for the study, **all** had lower levels of antibodies than the subjects who had never been vaccinated.

"Our study showed that a decreased immune response to some influenza strains may follow repeated annual vaccinations," Dannenberg said.

American medical organizations recommend annual flu shots for seniors since they consider them a "high risk" group. Flu is the fourth leading cause of death in this age group, they contend, although no figures are available to determine if the mortality rate is higher in those who have been vaccinated repeatedly.

SOURCE: "Annual flu shot for seniors debated," by Virginia Watson, Medical Tribune News Service, May 22, 1997.

Elderly face greater threat from pain relievers

The use of non-steroidal anti-inflammatory drugs (NSAIDs) among the elderly is associated with significant complications of serious digestive problems, according to a study at Emory University presented at the 62nd Annual Scientific Meeting of the American College of Gastroenterology in Chicago.

The commonly taken over-the-counter (OTC) pain relievers were found to cause gastroesophageal reflux disease, including peptic stricture, a narrowing or obstruction of the esophagus which can result from chronic acid injury and scarring of the lower esophagus.

A research team lead by gastroenterologist J. Patrick Waring, M.D. studied the relationship between age and complications of chronic acid reflux in a group of 79 individuals.

Patients were considered NSAID users if they had been taking low-dose aspirin, or prescription or OTC NSAIDS, more than twice a week for the previous six months. Patients over 65 were considered elderly.

Findings from endoscopic examination revealed that 28 patients (more than 35%) had esophageal stricture, and five experienced a narrowing of the esophagus called Schatzki's ring. Peptic stricture was significantly more common in elderly patients, and there was a greater likelihood of strictures in patients who took NSAIDS.

Statistical analysis showed that the older the person, the more likely the chance of getting peptic strictures, which are among the serious complications that can occur when acid reflux disease is not treated. Others include severe chest pain that can mimic a heart attack, bleeding, or a pre-malignant change in the lining of the esophagus called Barrett's esophagus.

This knowledge should make doctors less likely to prescribe or recommend NSAIDs to their older patients. However, a report published in the *Annuals of Internal Medicine* showed that frequently NSAIDs are prescribed unnecessarily and NSAID-related side effects are often inaccurately diagnosed and inappropriately managed.

A study of elderly patients conducted in Canada found that unnecessary NSAID prescriptions were written during 41.7% percent of office visits, and NSAIDS were prescribed even when patients had relative contraindications to NSAID therapy.

The study also showed that shorter office visits and failure to recognize contraindications to therapy seem to compromise the appropriateness of prescribing.

SOURCES: "Potential Complications from Common Pain Relievers More Likely in the Elderly," American College of Gastroenterology, November 2, 1997.

"Study Finds NSAIDS Often Prescribed Unnecessarily for Elderly Patients," *Annals of Internal Medicine,* September 15, 1997.

Drug companies target older population

At the beginning of this century, there were just slightly more than three million Americans over the age of sixty-five. At the start of the new century — less than three years away — there will be 35 million people in that category!

That figure has drug companies drooling in anticipation. To prepare, they have started development of 178 new drugs supposedly geared to "treating" age-related health problems.

That's in addition to the more than 400 drugs currently being tested for heart disease, cancer and stroke — the three leading killers of older Americans.

Although the industry brags about these new drugs, it fails to respond to criticism that few, if any, medications have been shown to actually cure a disease. In addition, they refuse to accept responsibility for — or even acknowledge the harmful and sometimes fatal side effects posed by — their products.

Yet, according to a Harvard research program, nearly a quarter of Americans 65 or older have been given prescriptions for drugs they probably shouldn't take.

The study, conducted by Dr. Steffi Woolhandler, found that more than 1.2 million Americans were taking diazepam, or *Valium*. This is a long-acting sedative that can cause grogginess and forgetfulness.

Many drugs that are over-prescribed are common ones, such as Valium, or dipyridamole, a blood thinner that the researchers say is worthless except for those with artificial heart valves. About 1.8 million Americans have prescriptions for dipyridamole. Only 98,000 Americans, half of them older than 65, received artificial heart valves in 1987, the last year for which figures were available.

The problem is so great that even the federal government got involved and issued a warning.

In 1995, the General Accounting Office — acting on a Congressional request — studied the situation and found that "the inappropriate prescription drug use is a serious health risk for the elderly, since they take more prescription drugs than other age groups, they often take several drugs at once, resulting in adverse drug reactions, and they do not efficiently eliminate drugs from their systems due to decreased body function."

Blame for improper use of these drugs wasn't dropped in the lap of the elderly patients, either. It was shared with physicians using outdated prescribing practices and pharmacists not performing drug utilization reviews.

SOURCES:"New Medicines in Development for Older Americans," Pharmaceutical Research and Manufacturers of America (PhRMA). Aug. 27, 1997.

"Inappropriate Drug Prescribing for the Community-Dwelling Elderly," by Sharon M. Wilcox, David U. Himmelstein, and Steffie Woolhandler. *Journal of the American Medical Association,* July 27, 1994.

"Prescription Drugs and the Elderly," General Accounting Office (GAO/HEHS-95-152), July 1995.

Reports of Alzheimer's progress called 'hype'

In a revealing expose carried by the *The New York Times* News Service, several prominent researchers accused their colleagues of deliberately misinforming the public about the lack of progress in treating or curing Alzheimer's disease.

According to Dr. Peter Davies, an Alzheimer's expert at the Albert Einstein College of Medicine in New York, "People have been playing the hype game a little too much." Such overstatements "may be good for funding, but I think it must be terrible for the public."

In the past few years, numerous Alzheimer's organizations, research centers, trust funds, and study groups have sprung up, turning the field into another profit-making industry competing for millions of dollars in research grant money. Medical scientists are flocking to the lucrative area of study — some 1,300 people attended an international Alzheimer's meeting in Japan this summer.

Now pharmaceutical companies are joining in the stampede, developing drugs to test for and treat the elusive ailment.

According to the Alzheimer's Association, four million Americans have been diagnosed with the disease, which translates into $90-$100 billion in yearly heath care costs.

Every few months — with increasing frequency it seems — newspaper headlines announce a new "breakthrough" that supposedly will put medicine another step closer to curing the disease. Yet, the truth is, medical science still hasn't even learned how to correctly diagnose Alzheimers. And, not only is there no known cure, even a successful treatment to slow its progression has yet to be found.

"Experts warn that much of the attention has been misguided," the wire service article noted. "They laugh in embarrassment at the scores of diagnostic tests that have been promoted over the years, each one hailed as a simple way to decide who has Alzheimer's disease and who does not. No test has yet been proved to be reliable."

SOURCE: "Hopes are rosy on Alzheimer's, but results slim," New York Times News Service, July 30, 1996.

Media distorts news about ibuprofen and Alzheimer's

The newspaper articles which appeared around the country early in 1997 had many people thinking that popping a pain killer every day could protect them from Alzheimer's disease. "Reduce risk by up to 60%" the reports exclaimed, adding that the information came from a research study published in the journal *Neurology.*

According to common media reports, taking frequent doses of the common anti-inflammatory drug ibuprofen over a two year period could reduce the risk of getting the disease.

But the media downplayed the "bad news" contained in the actual research report, including a warning by the researchers themselves that widespread use of ibuprofen could do more harm than good. "Ibuprofen can shut down your kidneys," stated researcher Dr. Claudia Kawas of the Johns Hopkins School of Medicine. "That would be a terrible thing to do while trying to prevent something you might not even get."

To their credit, the researchers also tried to warn the media and the public that their study was not to be considered definitive, particularly since it was based on information provided by patients rather than clinical research.

"We will need clinical trials to prove that (it) confers protection and, ultimately, to make public health recommendations to reduce risk," stated co-researcher Dr. Walter Stewart, also of Johns Hopkins.

SOURCE: "Risk of Alzheimer's disease and duration of NSAID use," by Walter Stewart, Claudia Kawas, et. al. *Neurology,* March 1997.

Benefits of mammograms for elders disputed

A panel of experts at the National Institutes of Health (NIH) Consensus Development Conference has declared there is no proof that the potential benefits of mammograms outweigh the risks involved for women under 50 years-old.

A number of "cancer societies" argued, saying the tests — which cost between $50-200 each - - are a necessity for all women over 40, despite the fact that radiation from yearly mammograms during ages 40-49 has been estimated to cause one additional breast cancer death per 10,000 women.

Now, another study has uncovered that many women are still being subjected to the controversial test after age 75 — a practice which researchers say has "limited" benefits.

At the American Geriatric Society's annual conference in Atlanta, the Masonic Geriatric Healthcare Center released the results of its study examining the value of mammography screening for women aged 75 and older who had no history of breast cancer.

Data gathered suggested that, when effects of treatment preferences and co-morbidities were considered, the overall value of screening mammography was limited in this population. While the risk of developing breast cancer increases with age and accounts for two percent of all deaths among women over 80, there have been very few studies assessing the risks and benefits of screening older women.

In this study, 384 mammograms were administered to 182 women over the age of 75 who did not have a history of breast cancer. Initial examinations produced abnormal findings for more than 48% of the study population. Yet, only 13 were later diagnosed as actually having breast cancer. Of these, just seven chose treatment, while five refused due to co-existing diseases (one decision was still pending when the study results were released).

One of the patients receiving treatment died of congestive heart failure, and two of those refusing treatment died, one secondary to heart disease. Only one patient died as a result of breast cancer. Nearly all patients in the sample study (96%) had some form of written advanced directive in their charts.

According to Masonic Geriatric Healthcare Center's Vice President of Medical Affairs Erlinda Rauch, M.D., who administered the study with her colleagues Ronald Schwartz, M.D., and Gerard Kerins, M.D., "One of the greatest drawbacks of screening women of this age is the anxiety an abnormal mammogram can cause. Considering that 3.85% of the study group was treated, the overall value of mammography screening was limited in this study."

Although American Cancer Society guidelines call for annual mammography screening for women beginning at age 40, there is no upper age limit specified. Considering that the number of women in the 75-plus age category continues to grow rapidly, along with pressure to provide cost-effective care, it stands to reason that further research is necessary in order to establish appropriate care guidelines, said the researchers.

SOURCE: "Value of Mammography for Women Aged 75+," by Masonic Geriatric Healthcare Center, May 17, 1997. Presented at the American Geriatric Society's annual conference in Atlanta.

Medications increase car accident rate in elderly

Older people taking a certain type of drug for anxiety or insomnia are at increased risk for motor vehicle crashes, according to an article in the *Journal of the American Medical Association (JAMA)*.

Brenda Hemmelgarn, M.N., Samy Suissa, Ph.D., and colleagues from McGill University and Royal Victoria Hospital, Montreal, Quebec, studied 224,734 drivers, aged 67 to 84 years, to determine if benzodiazepines are associated with car crashes in elderly drivers.

The researchers found a 45% increased rate of motor vehicle crashes involving injuries for elderly patients during the first seven days of taking a long-acting form of benzodiazepine. After continuous use of the drug for up to one year, the increased risk was twenty-six percent.

Benzodiazepines are among the most frequently prescribed medications for the elderly. Side effects include drowsiness, sedation, confusion and impaired motor function, according to information cited in the study.

The authors noted: "Although evidence from randomized trials is not available, our findings, in combination with other recent studies of benzodiazepine use in the elderly, indicate a significant risk of injurious motor vehicle crash associated with long-half-life products. The risk appears to be highest within the first seven days of initiating therapy and is reduced significantly but remains elevated with prolonged use."

They also wrote: "In the present study we found that risk remained elevated for continuous use of up to one year, contrary to what has been previously speculated. These results suggest that tolerance to the sedative and psychomotor effects of these long-half-life products may not develop with continued use, or, as has been proposed, tolerance may develop for some but not all of the psychomotor skills."

In an accompanying editorial in the same issue of *JAMA*, Wayne A. Ray, Ph.D., from Vanderbilt University School of Medicine, Nashville, Tenn., wrote: "The studies of benzodiazepines and crash involvement add to the already long list of reasons to avoid benzodiazepines in older patients — particularly long-half-life drugs or long-term use ... Even if short-acting benzodiazepines are less likely to increase the risk of injuries, other adverse effects suggest these agents be used very cautiously among elderly patients."

Dr. Ray continued: "Yet, benzodiazepine use is but one of many factors that may impair driving and that are more common among older than younger drivers ... It seems unavoidable that growing numbers of functionally impaired drivers will trigger public concern with safety and perhaps even attempts to more tightly regulate driving among the elderly. Given the nearly complete reliance on driving for mobility in most of the United States, such restrictions could severely compromise older persons' independence."

"Unfortunately, research on crash epidemiology in the elderly is in its infancy and the times are not [favorable] for funding major new research initiatives," Ray concluded. "Nevertheless, absent a reinvigorated research agenda for crashes in older drivers, we are unlikely to strike the delicate balance between safe driving and the mobility and independence of an aging population."

SOURCE: *The Journal of the American Medical Association (JAMA)* 278;1997:27-31.

New arthritis treatment increases risk, lacks long-term benefits

Doctors touting a new, stronger drug regimen for rheumatoid arthritis are failing to emphasize that the effect of the drug combination wears off just months after patients stop taking it.

According to a report in the British medical journal, *The Lancet,* the new therapy consists of using a combination of sulfasalazine, the steroid prednisolone, and methotrexate.

Although patients subjected to this combination reported a decrease in the joint degeneration associated with the disease, the benefit was only temporary. As soon as they stopped taking the drug, the benefits stopped, and after 10 months, they were no better off than the group given less toxic chemical therapy.

"By the end of the study the patients had reverted to the same level of disease activity as that in the group treated by sulfasalazine alone," said Dr. Paul Emery in an editorial in the same issue. "The therapy was effective during the time it was prescribed but had no impact on the underlying disease process or activity."

The short term benefits appear to be greatly outweighed by the increased risk of side effects posed by long term use of the drug combination, which can include bone-thinning.

SOURCE: *The Lancet,* August 4, 1997.

Chapter 5

The "miracle of antibiotics

W hen antibiotics were first developed, they were considered a "miracle" drug because they seemed to be able to aid the body in fighting
off infections and invading bacteria. The drugs actually were helpful
for some people with weakened immune systems who needed outside intervention to get through immediate and acute health crises.

But even a "miracle" can be abused.

Medical doctors started prescribing the drugs after nearly every office visit
— even for conditions that couldn't be helped at all by antibiotics. They
pumped the drug into our systems and now, decades later, we're paying the
price with antibiotic-resistant super- bacteria and impaired natural antibody
functions. Tragically, despite warnings from the World Health Organization
and more progressive health care experts, M.D.s still rely heavily on the drugs.

United Nations' leader blames spread
of disease on overuse of antibiotics

The annual report issued by the World Health Organization (WHO) warned
that the spread of many devastating diseases — including AIDS and Ebola —
may be blamed in great part on the overuse of antibiotics throughout the
world. The report was issued after the WHO convened its 49th annual session
in the Palais des Nations, Geneva, from 20-25 May 1996.

According to WHO Director-General Dr. Hiroshi Nakajima, "The optimism
of a relatively few years ago that many of these diseases could be brought
under control has led to a fatal complacency. This complacency is now costing
millions of lives."

The report listed several other critical factors, including poverty and overcrowding, but singled out "the uncontrolled and inappropriate use of antibiotics," as one of the primary reasons for the outbreak of drug-resistant strains
of infectious diseases.

"They are used by too many people to treat the wrong kind of infections at
the wrong dosage and for the wrong period of time," the report states. The
overuse of antibiotics has been shown to weaken the body's natural immune
system.

*SOURCES:*World Health Report 1996, World Health Organization, Geneva,
Switzerland, May 1996.

More evidence of antibiotic overuse

Amoxicillin and other antibiotics are frequently used to prevent recurrent middle ear infections that affect 15% of America's children.

But a study supported by the Agency for Health Care Policy and Research indicated that use of these antibiotics may not be a good idea.

The study showed that children with recurrent middle ear infections — that is, three infections within six months or four in a year — fare about the same as children given a placebo, with 61-64% remaining free of new infections during the study period.

Also, researchers say that the excessive antibiotic use, which has the potential to promote acquisition of antibiotic-resistant bacterial pneumonia, already is becoming more prevalent.

SOURCES: "Continuous twice daily or once daily amoxicillin prophylaxis compared with placebo for children with recurrent acute otitis media," *Pediatric Infectious Disease Journal 16.*

"Amoxicillin is Often Prescribed to Prevent Middle Ear Infections in Young Children, But it is Only Marginally Effective," Agency for Health Care Policy and Research, Sept. 29, 1997.

Medical journal repeats antibiotic fears

A scientific literature review published in the *New England Journal of Medicine (NEJM)* has added more evidence about the dangers of overuse and misuse of antibiotics.

According to researchers Drs. Howard S. Gold and Robert C. Moellering Jr., antibiotics seemed to be true "wonder drugs" when they were first discovered. "However," they explained in their *NEJM* paper, "it was soon evident that bacterial pathogens were unlikely to surrender unconditionally, because some pathogens rapidly became resistant to many of the first effective drugs."

Each time the bacteria becomes resistent to the existing antibiotic, the response has been to develop a new one. "Unfortunately, there is no assurance that the development of new antimicrobial drugs can keep pace with the ability of bacterial pathogens to develop resistance," the report warns.

In essence, the medical profession — through its use of antibiotics — has bred numerous "super bacteria" which are resistant to many of the current antibiotics. The adaptability of the bacteria makes it nearly impossible to create drugs that will stop them. In fact, new drugs are more likely to breed even stronger, more resilient bacteria.

Health officials all over the world are fearful that the new superbacteria — combined with human immune systems which have been weakened through reliance on artificial antibiotics - - are responsible for outbreaks of epidemics such as AIDS and ebola.

And, the problem is not confined to third-world countries.

"Overuse and inappropriate use of these drugs are hardly unique to these countries," stated the researchers.

"A recent survey by the Centers for Disease Control and Prevention documented increasing use of broader-spectrum, more expensive antimicrobial drugs by office-based physicians in the United States to treat otitis media, sinusitis, and other common infections. The widespread use of antimicrobial drugs for immunocompromised patients and in the intensive care units of modern hospitals clearly results in the selection of the multidrug-resistant organisms that cause serious nosocomial infections."

A situation reported in California is a good example of the problem cited in the *NEJM* report. Officials at the UC Davis Medical Center reported that, within a two-week period, 10 patients contracted an infection from the enterococcus bacteria, a normally harmless bacteria commonly found in the stomach.

More frightening, however, was the fact that the bacteria appears to have developed a resistance to vancomycin, the antibiotic usually used to treat it. As of 1994, the Center's doctors had never seen a case of the infection which did not respond to vancomycin. In 1995, UC Davis and several other Sacramento hospitals all reported at least one case.

The 10 patients made up the largest reported hospital cluster ever seen in the county.

SOURCES: "Drug Therapy: Antimicrobial-Drug Resistance," by Howard S. Gold, and Robert C. Moellering Jr., *New England Journal of Medicine,* Nov. 7, 1996.

"Normally mild bacterial infection found to be resistant to all antibiotics," Scripps-McClatchy Western, October 28, 1996.

M.D.s still prescribing unneeded antibiotics

Many physicians prescribe antibiotic drugs for three common respiratory illnesses although the drugs do little or nothing to treat the problems, according to an article which appeared in the Sept. 17, 1997 issue of *The Journal of the American Medical Association (JAMA).*

Ralph Gonzales, M.D., M.S.P.H., from the University of Colorado Health Sciences Center in Denver, and his colleagues conducted the study, measuring how often antibiotic prescriptions are given to adult patients in the United States. They were trying to figure out why some medical doctors continue to pass out the drugs despite numerous warnings in recent years about the overuse of antibiotics.

The researchers found that, in patients who sought medical attention for colds, upper respiratory tract infections or bronchitis, 50 to 70% were given prescriptions for antibiotics. In fact, office visits for colds, upper respiratory tract infections and bronchitis resulted in approximately 12 million antibiotic prescriptions, accounting for 21% of all antibiotic prescriptions to adults in 1992.

The authors noted that these illnesses are most commonly caused by viruses — and antibiotic drugs are of "little or no benefit" in those cases!

Frequent use of antibiotics can cause bacteria to become resistant to antibiotic drugs, a potentially dangerous situation.

"The increasing prevalence of resistant organisms has been attributed, at least in part, to high rates of antibiotic prescribing, not all of which is necessary," according to Margaret A. Winker, M.D., *JAMA* senior editor.

The researchers also found that women and patients in rural areas of the United States were more likely than other groups to be prescribed antibiotics for the three viral illnesses, whereas African-Americans were less likely to be given antibiotic prescriptions. Factors that had no bearing on the rate of antibiotic prescriptions were patient age, patients being of Hispanic origin, geographic region, physician specialty and sources of payment.

The authors acknowledged that getting medical doctors to discontinue the dangerous (although lucrative) practice of prescribing unnecessary antibiotics won't be easy.

"Decreasing unnecessary antibiotic use to combat the emergence of antibiotic-resistant bacteria in our communities will be a difficult task," they admitted.

In an editorial published in the same issue, Benjamin Schwartz, M.D., and colleagues from the Centers for Disease Control and Prevention in Atlanta, noted that "unrealistic patient expectations coupled with insufficient time to discuss with patients why an antibiotic is not needed" are the major reasons why physicians over-prescribe antibiotic drugs when they know the drugs will be ineffective.

However, they also conceded that, "Although less readily admitted, physicians' inadequate knowledge of the spectrum of symptoms and signs and the natural history of respiratory illnesses also contributes to antibiotic overuse."

SOURCE: The Journal of the American Medical Association, Sept. 17, 1997.

Most infants given antibiotics during first six months of life

Despite repeated warnings about the over-use and misuse of antibiotics, doctors continue to pump the drugs into our nation's children at an alarming rate.

One medical study showed that 70% of all infants in the U.S. are subjected to their first course of antibiotics during the first 200 days of their lives. Researchers found that otitis media (middle-ear infection) was the most common reason for antibiotic treatment in infants and *amoxicillin* was the antibiotic most often prescribed.

However, in recent years more and more health care professionals have warned that the misuse of antibiotics as a "line of first defense" has not only weakened the natural immune system but created a variety of "superbacteria" which are resistant to any antibiotics.

Early in 1996, the United Nations World Health Organization published its annual report and blamed the misuse of antibiotics for many of the new epidemics arising throughout the world, including AIDS and ebola.

The report listed several other critical factors, including poverty and overcrowding, but singled out "the uncontrolled and inappropriate use of antibiotics," as one of the primary reasons for the outbreak of drug-resistant strains of infectious diseases.

An investigative report into the use of antibiotics noted: "A child's ear infection offers a classic example of how over-treatment with antibiotics can lead to the development of drug- resistant strains of bacteria. For years, amoxicillin — a penicillin-like antibiotic — was the standard treatment for acute otitis media. However, these infections usually clear, without treatment, in two to three days."

This report, published in *Ladies Home Journal* also noted that "because amoxicillin has been so overprescribed, some ear infections that in the past might have responded to it no longer do. As a result, doctors are forced to prescribe one after another of stronger — and more expensive — medications. Furthermore, the stronger antibiotics are the broad-spectrum ones, which kill the so-called good bacteria as well as the bad, making children vulnerable to secondary infections."

SOURCES: "Antibiotic Use During the First 200 Days of Life," by George R. Bergus, M.D., et. al., *Archives of Family Medicine,* October 1996, pps. 523- 526.

World Health Report 1996, World Health Organization, Geneva, Switzerland, May 1996.

"A spoonful of medicine: unnecessary drugs are not only useless, they have the potential to seriously harm our children," by Margery D. Rosen. *Ladies Home Journal,* April 1995.

MDs blame parents for antibiotic abuse in children

Despite a growing concern over "antibiotic resistance," pediatricians continue to unnecessarily prescribe antibiotics for children. Yet, a study published by the American Academy of Pediatrics on Pediatrics electronic pages, says the parents are to blame.

According to the article, pediatricians give these harmful and unnecessary drugs to children because parents demand them. Ironically, the study also faulted parents for giving their children antibiotics **without** seeking physician advice — even though it acknowledged that physicians will often prescribe the drugs anyway, merely because the patient requests them.

Researchers from Boston Medical Center, Boston, surveyed 400 parents and 61 pediatricians and found 18% of parents give their children antibiotics without consulting a physician.

Nine out of 10 thought antibiotics were needed for ear infections, eight out of 10 thought antibiotics were needed for throat infections, and six out of 10 thought antibiotics were needed for cough and fever.

"Growing bacterial resistance to antibiotics represents a global threat to the health of the world's population," the authors stated. "If parents can better understand the role of antibiotics in the treatment of disease, they may exert less pressure on physicians to dispense antibiotics inappropriately."

The study focused its criticism on the parents rather than on the doctors who often fail to act in their patients' best interest by failing to educate parents rather than provide drugs on demand.

SOURCE: "Parents Unnecessarily Request Antibiotics," American Academy of Pediatrics, Pediatrics electronic pages. June 2, 1997.

Antibiotics over-prescribed in bronchitis cases

Antibiotics — once thought of as a "miracle drug" — took yet another hit when a researcher found that antibiotic use in treating bronchitis is unnecessary and risky.

"Clinicians often prescribe antibiotics to treat acute bronchitis despite scant evidence that this approach is effective," stated Dr. William Hueston, University of Wisconsin-Madison Medical School Department of Family Medicine, Eau Claire, in *The Journal of Family Practice*.

Bronchitis, which is an inflammation of the linings of the major lung airways, can cause persistent cough as well as difficulty breathing and other discomfort. Many medical doctors continue to use antibiotics as a treatment, despite proof that acute bronchitis is usually triggered by viral infections — which do not respond to antibiotics.

Surprisingly, Dr. Hueston tried to put at least part of the blame on patients themselves when he said, "Evidence suggests that physicians may prescribe antibiotics because of an expectation that the patient wants an antibiotic."

Such a conclusion would seem illogical since Hueston himself admitted that routine prescriptions for antibiotics "increase the (medical) cost per episode by about 16%," even with the use of relatively cheap antibiotics such as erythromycin.

In fact, he added that he wondered "whether patients are willing to pay this extra cost for a small chance of quicker relief from their cough or to avoid the inconvenience of having to return to the physician if their cough persists."

If antibiotics were merely expensive placebos, the continued use of them for bronchitis and other viral infections might not be as worrisome. However, as Hueston pointed out, "Growing concerns about increasing antimicrobial resistance presumably linked to antibiotic overuse indicate that re-evaluation of the use of antibiotics... may be warranted."

Doctors who try to justify their prescriptions for antibiotics by saying "the patient wanted them," can solve the problem with patient education and explanations. Once they understand the facts, Hueston said, patients remain "satisfied with their care," even when antibiotics are not prescribed.

Although about 5-10% of bronchitis cases are caused by a bacteria and not a virus, and therefore might possibly respond to antibiotics, the test needed to determine this is expensive and inaccurate, Hueston pointed out.

He believes the best way to treat bronchitis is the wait-and-see approach. Most cases of bronchitis are "self-limited" and resolve themselves in a few weeks.

SOURCE: *The Journal of Family Practice*, 1997; 44(3):261-265.

Antibiotics do not improve
sinusitis symptoms, study shows

Primary care physicians (family doctors) commonly prescribe antibiotics to treat acute maxillary sinusitis (inflamed membranes of the sinuses), although there is no evidence that this approach is effective.

A report in the British medical journal *The Lancet* found that antibiotics did nothing more than the placebos used as the control.

Study subjects were all referred by family doctors who thought antibiotic treatment was called for because of the severity of the symptoms. The patients were given either antibiotics or a placebo and the progress of their symptoms (headache, increase of pain in the face on bending, nasal obstruction, and nasal discharge) was checked by ear, nose, and throat specialists after one and two weeks.

All patients were also asked to report to their doctors any relapses that occurred during the year following treatment.

After two weeks, the results for the two groups were similar. Symptoms had greatly improved or disappeared in 83% of the antibiotic group and in 77% of the placebo group, which was not considered a significant difference.

One year after treatment, the number of relapses did not differ significantly between the patients treated with antibiotics and those treated with placebo.

Although this report merely confirms what other researchers have found in the past, medical doctors continue to treat patients with antibiotics. In recent years, the over-use of antibiotics has been the cause of major deterioration in human immune system responses and, according to the World Health Organization, may be a direct cause of the outbreak of worldwide epidemics such as Ebola and even AIDS.

SOURCES: The Lancet, March 8, 1997.

World Health Report 1996, World Health Organization, Geneva, Switzerland, May 1996.

Antibiotic found to cause
tendon inflammation, damage

The medical misuse and overuse of antibiotics has been implicated in the development of several "superbacteria," as well as the outbreak of new epidemics and diseases around the world.

Health experts are expressing concern about another risk posed by a class of antibiotics known as fluoroquinolones — often used to treat bladder, respiratory and other infections. According to reports from both American and European researchers, the drug can inflame and even rupture patients tendons.

In July 1996, the health advocacy group Public Citizen filed a petition with the Food and Drug Administration (FDA) to force manufacturers of fluoroquinolone antibiotics to put a warning about the danger on the drug's label.

The group cited 130 reports of tendon inflammation or rupture in people who used the prescription drug in England, France and Belgium. About 14.4 million prescriptions for fluoroquinolones were filled in the United States in a single year.

"Doctors and the public must be warned to immediately discontinue use of fluoroquinolone antibiotics at the first sign of tendon pain," Public Citizen Director Dr. Sidney Wolfe stated during a press conference.

The FDA had received at least 52 reports of patients in the U.S. who have suffered tendon damage. In the past, the labels warned against using fluoroquinolones in children, adolescents, and pregnant or lactating women.

But Public Citizen said that warning isn't strong enough.

"Doctors and the public must be warned to immediately discontinue use of fluoroquinolone antibiotics at the first sign of tendon pain," Dr. Wolfe stressed, adding that continuing the drug after the tendons become sore can cause them to rupture. Most of the ruptures occur in the Achilles tendon and may require surgery.

*SOURCES:*Media release, Public Citizen. August 1, 1996.

"Fluoroquinolone-Associated Tendon Rupture," *New England Journal of Medicine*. 1995;332:193.

Antibiotic treatment does not help sore throat

The scenario takes place every day all over the world. A person with a sore throat goes to a medical doctor. After the pre-requisite command for the patient to "say aah" while the doctor peers down a red, irritated throat, he or she hands over a prescription for penicillin or some other antibiotic.

That may be the worst thing the doctor can do, according to a research study published in the *British Medical Journal*. Prescribing antibiotics for sore throat has only marginal benefit and makes the growing problem of antibiotic-resistant bacteria even greater.

In a randomized trial of three approaches to sore throat — a 10 day prescription of antibiotics, no antibiotics, and a delayed prescription if the sore throat had not begun to improve after three days — the authors found there was no difference between the three groups in the incidence of complications.

Partly because of air pollution and other environmental factors, respiratory conditions have increased greatly in recent years and more people are trying to find medical solutions to the problem. In fact, in Britain, the number of people visiting doctors because of sore throats and related health complaints has increased by 14% in 10 years.

Yet, there's nothing medical doctors can do that the human body can't do by itself, given time. According to the researchers, the average duration of a sore throat is five days and almost 40% of people have a sore throat for longer than this — with or without antibiotics.

SOURCE: British Medical Journal, No 7104 Volume 315, August 9, 1997.

Chapter 6

For the sake of our children

Next to our elderly, our children are in the greatest danger from the medical mindset so prevalent in this country. We all want what's best for our kids, and we've been brainwashed to believe that this means pumping drugs into them from the moment they're born. The belief that medicine is needed to ensure health in children is so strong that parents have actually been accused of child abuse because they refused to allow their children to be subjected to the risks of vaccines, medications and other invasive medical procedures.

Most children are born into this world with perfectly healthy bodies, which innately "know" how to maintain the highest level of health possible. They have the right chemicals, in the right amounts, to function properly in this world. Yet, medical science is arrogant enough to think it can improve on the original design and immediately bombards that body with dangerous and sometimes potentially deadly chemicals. The result is not improved function, but impaired function. That tiny body not only has to adapt to its environment, it now has to assimilate foreign chemicals in its system.

Infants, toddlers, adolescents and teens are all subjected to the same treatment with the obvious result that childhood health problems are soaring. Chronic ear infections, asthma, childhood diabetes, and "new" diseases like attention deficit disorder, are all at epidemic proportions and getting worse. The reliance on medical treatment hasn't helped at all, yet parents are reluctant to reject it for a better way, and the medical and drug industries continue to hide the truth from them.

The drugging of America's kids

Lacy Keele was just five-years old when she died of a drug overdose. She wasn't one of those lost children we read about barely out of the cradle and already addicted to heroin or cocaine. She merely had a cold and her mother thought it was safe to treat the symptoms with Tylenol.

It wasn't.

Lacy's liver shut down and she died — making her another statistic on the list of many children who are inadvertently poisoned each year with common over-the-counter (OTC) remedies and prescription medicines.

This is a new kind of drug abuse epidemic which is threatening the lives and health of hundreds of thousands of American children. Well-meaning parents are believing the lies told to them by medical doctors and drug makers and are pumping their kids full of toxic substances — many of which are specifically marketed to children!

The three main areas of concern are common cold medications, including aspirin and non- aspirin pain relievers such as Tylenol; antibiotics; and behavior modification drugs like Ritalin and Prozac.

Colds and flu

Almost all surveys conducted in this country have revealed that *at least* half of all children **routinely** receive either OTC or prescription drugs, particularly for common childhood ailments, colds and flu.

One such study, published in the *Journal of the American Medical Association (JAMA)*, found that more than 50% of all mothers surveyed had given their 3-year-olds an OTC medication, primarily Tylenol or cough or cold medicines, in the prior 30 days.

The researchers questioned the wisdom of this action.

"The use of cough and cold medicines is increasingly being called into question due to the striking absence of efficacy data on cough and cold medicines in children," they pointed out. "The efficacy of cough and cold medications was the focus of a congressional hearing, during which the chairman commented: 'The sad fact is, much of the billion-dollar cold medication industry may be based more on hype than on health care.'

"Viewed from this perspective," they noted, "the high use rate of these medications may be a tremendous waste of money and may unnecessarily expose children to toxicity."

Another study noted that two-thirds of all families kept their medicine cabinets stocked with at least four and as many as eight different nonprescription drugs for their kids!

Even the Food & Drug Administration (FDA) — which seldom protests anything the pharmaceutical or medical industries do — has voiced concern with the over-medicating of our children.

"Before parents dole out OTC drugs, they should consider whether they're truly necessary," stated Paula Botstein, M.D., pediatrician and acting director of the FDA's Office of Drug Evaluation III. "Americans love to medicate — perhaps too much."

An FDA consumer report also noted, "Not every cold needs medicine. Common viruses run their course in seven to 10 days with or without medication. While some OTC medications can sometimes make children more comfortable and help them eat and rest better, others may trigger allergic reactions or changes for the worse in sleeping, eating and behavior. Antibiotics, available by prescription, don't work at all on cold viruses."

Botstein added, "There's not a medicine to cure everything or to make every symptom go away. Just because your child is miserable and your heart aches to see her that way, doesn't mean she needs drugs."

Her sentiments were echoed by the *JAMA* study researchers.

"Although they may be annoying or worrisome to the parent," they noted that "the signs of upper respiratory tract infection, particularly cough, may not be distressing to the child, in which case it is truly the parent administering the OTC medication who is being 'treated.'"

Antibiotics

Another type of drug that is grossly over-prescribed to children is antibiotics. Not only — as the researchers stated — are antibiotics useless on cold viruses, but they have literally decimated the human immune system and given rise to a whole new generation of super-bacteria.

"In the last twenty-five years, the miracle of antibiotics has boomeranged," stated Stuart B. Levy, M.D., professor of medicine and molecular biology at Tufts University School of Medicine, in Boston, and author of "The Antibiotic Paradox: How Miracle Drugs are Destroying the Miracle."

He explained that, "The list of antibiotics that are no longer effective in treating illnesses — everything from ear, skin and urinary tract infections to pneumonia, tuberculosis and malaria — is long and unparalleled. And this lack of response is due, in large measure, to the overuse and misuse of these antibiotics."

The World Health Organization agrees.

In its 1996 report, the WHO singled out "the uncontrolled and inappropriate use of antibiotics," as one of the primary reasons for the outbreak of drug-resistant strains of infectious diseases. "They are used by too many people to treat the wrong kind of infections at the wrong dosage and for the wrong period of time," the report stated.

Yet, despite the numerous warnings, many doctors continue to prescribe antibiotics to most of their patients.

A report in *Ladies Home Journal* noted, "A child's ear infection offers a classic example of how over-treatment with antibiotics can lead to the development of drug-resistant strains of bacteria. For years, amoxicillin — a penicillin-like antibiotic — was the standard treatment for acute otitis media. However, these infections usually clear, without treatment, in two to three days. ...

"However," the *Journal* report continued," because amoxicillin has been so overprescribed, some ear infections that in the past might have responded to it no longer do. As a result, doctors are forced to prescribe one after another of stronger — and more expensive — medications. Furthermore, the stronger antibiotics are the broad-spectrum ones, which kill the so-called good bacteria as well as the bad, making children vulnerable to secondary infections."

"So far," said Dr. Levy, "we've been able to stay a step ahead of most drug-resistant bacteria by creating newer, more powerful drugs. But for how much longer? Every person taking an antibiotic potentially contributes a little bit to the environmental pool of resistant bacteria."

Behavioral drugs

By far the most controversial medications being prescribed for children are the behavioral modification drugs such as Ritalin and Prozac. Although many health care professionals have expressed deep concern about both the short-term and long-term effects of these powerful drugs, medical doctors continue to prescribe them at a record-breaking pace.

The increase in the use of anti-depressants and stimulants for children is staggering. In the past two years alone, prescriptions for children on antide-pressants (including Prozac, Zoloft and Paxil) have risen almost eighty percent. Today, more than 1.3 million children are being drugged up on these medicines. The growth rate in prescribing for children is three times faster than for adults!

The increase in the use of Ritalin — primarily for hyperactivity — is just as astonishing.

Since 1990, the production of Ritalin has quadrupled. By 1994, in excess of eight TONS was being prescribed each year! Some 1.5 million children are tak-ing it on a regular basis — more than two-and-a-half times the number who received it just five years ago.

Even though experts say that most children are not being properly diag-nosed and that doses are merely guesswork since no clinical trials have been conducted on children, prescriptions are still being written as fast as doctors can reach for their pens.

When will it stop?

The key phrase of the medical doctor's Hippocratic Oath is "Do No Harm," yet it is obvious that the overuse and abuse of prescription drugs continues — despite the harm it does to our nation's children.

Compounding the crime, the pharmaceutical industry relentlessly pumps out drugs which are marketed directly at children, often using marketing tech-niques which exploit a parent's sense of guilt or helplessness.

There's no question that the madness must stop before we destroy the future health of an entire generation.

"It is well documented that the average American doctor is writing too many prescriptions, and most are ineffective, needlessly expensive, possibly dangerous," stated Ray Woosley, M.D., Ph.D., professor and chairman of phar-macology at Georgetown University Medical School, in Washington, D.C.

Yet, it seems unlikely that the change will come from the medical community — and it definitely will not be championed by the drug makers. That means par-ents must learn to "just say no" to unnecessary over-the-counter and prescription drugs. If they aren't the ones to do it, their children will remain unprotected from those who apparently are willing to let them die rather than sacrifice profit.

SOURCES: "Over-the-counter medication use among U.S. preschool-age children," *The Journal of the American Medical Association,* Oct. 5, 1994 v272 n13 p1025(6).

"Rational use of over-the-counter medications in young children," by Anne Godomski. *The Journal of the American Medical Association,* Oct. 5, 1994 v272 n13 p1063(2).

"The Right Stuff For Our Kids?" by Susan Sachs. *Newsday,* June 6, 1996.

"How to give medicine to children," by Rebecca D. Williams, *FDA Consumer,* Jan.-Feb. 1996 v30 n1 p6(4).

"World Health Report 1996," World Health Organization, Geneva, Switzerland, May 1996.

"Doing more good than harm with children's medications," by Stephen J. Ackerman. *FDA Consumer,* March 1989 v23 n2 p28(4).

"A spoonful of medicine: unnecessary drugs are not only useless, they have the potential to seriously harm our children," by Margery D. Rosen. *Ladies Home Journal,* April 1995 v112 n4 p122(5).

Doctors "guess" at drug doses for kids

When President Bill Clinton announced that in the future, drug makers would be expected to conduct tests to determine whether their medications are safe and effective for children, many parents were surprised. They had not realized that more than half of all medications widely given to children have never been tested to make sure they are safe for them.

The presidential announcement brought to light what some see as a shameful indictment of the drug and medical industries, two multi-billion dollar conglomerates which are more interested in profit than in the lives of our world's children.

Because of the lack of tests, doctors often guess at dosages, exposing children to toxic amounts of drugs.

The problem is not only in the amount of the drug, but in the affect of the drug on a child's body. Because of differences in size, physiology, temperament and metabolism, children cannot be considered merely as small adults and given a reduced portion of an adult drug.

In making his announcement, Mr. Clinton referred to a case in which doctors gave infants reduced doses of adult antibiotics. Later, it was discovered that the drug accumulates in children's livers — 23 of the babies died.

In 1994, the drug industry — faced with regulations which would have required testing and proper labeling — managed to walk away with an agreement to "voluntarily" comply with the proposed demands. They failed to take any steps in that direction and, in the past five years, less 25% of all drugs approved in the U.S. have been tested for children.

The drug companies argue that such testing is too expensive.

According to White House spokespeople, testing the 10 drugs which should be tested immediately — including drugs often given to children for asthma and depression — would cost $10-20 million. Drug companies routinely gross billions of dollars each year on these drugs.

"In 1994, over 3 million prescriptions for five drugs were prescribed to children without adequate studies being conducted on their safety and effectiveness. These include drugs for treating asthma, depression and nausea," said Dr. Sidney Wolfe, Director of Public Citizen's Health Research Group.

Another danger for children is the "off label" use of drugs, that is, the use of drugs for ailments other than the ones which the drug was tested for.

Under an amendment to one bill which was working its way through Congress in 1997, drug companies would be allowed to promote off-label uses of their products by sending articles from medical journals to doctors. "Such wholesale promotion of off-label usage exposes children to potentially dangerous drugs," charged Wolfe.

SOURCES: White House Press Conference, August 13, 1997.

"Doublespeak: Clinton administration announces new testing requirements on medicine for children but supports legislation allowing "off-label" drug promotion," Media Advisory, Public Citizen's Health Research Group, August 13, 1997.

Aspirin and children: A deadly combination

The story was so frightening that it could have come from a Robin Cook novel or a made-for-television disaster movie. Normal, healthy children in the process of getting over routine childhood illnesses such as chicken pox or the flu are suddenly hit with a string of symptoms: vomiting, irritability, tiredness. They slip into a coma, battling for their lives.

But it wasn't a film, it was a real-life nightmare. In 1977, it happened to nearly 2,300 children and nearly one third of them died.

And it wasn't some strange disease or microbe that killed them — it was aspirin.

When children are given aspirin during a variety of viral infections (including chicken pox, mumps, German measles, measles, mononucleosis, herpes simplex and even the flu) they risk developing a condition known as Reye's Syndrome (also called RS) after the Australian doctor who first realized what was causing the deaths.

Tragically, the medical profession knew about the link between aspirin and RS years before those 2,300 children were stricken. The syndrome was first described by Dr. R. Reye in the early 1960s and the fact that it was caused by aspirin was suggested by research as early as 1962.

Even though the Centers for Disease Control (CDC) had RS "under surveillance" from 1973-76, they did nothing to warn the public. While they stood by and watched, as many as 550 cases of RS were reported each year to the CDC, and probably many other cases went unreported because of misdiagnosis. Whenever there was a major outbreak of influenza A, the number of cases rose, and at its worst, fatality rates reached forty percent.

But RS doesn't just strike children. It can be just as devastating in teenagers and even some adults — and the cause is still aspirin.

Despite mounting evidence, the makers and marketers of aspirin refused to admit their drug could be killing so many children.

According to an in-depth report that appeared in *The Milbank Quarterly,* drug companies immediately began issuing reports which contradicted the research results.

"Their earliest efforts were to critically evaluate the case-control studies, and to publish reports questioning their conclusiveness," the *Milbank* report noted.

"In March 1982," it continued, "Plough, Inc. sent letters to pediatricians questioning the validity of reports and news stories linking aspirin to RS and recommending continued prescribing of aspirin for the reduction of fever in children. Other industry-sponsored reports were published as articles or letters in medical journals. For example, the June 1982 issue of *Pediatrics* contained an industry-sponsored report suggesting that early symptoms of RS preceded and precipitated increased aspirin use in children later diagnosed with RS."

Although it dragged its feet for nearly a decade, the Food & Drug Administration finally decided to warn the public about the risk, and, in 1983, prepared a brochure that was to be distributed to grocery stores where parents commonly bought the drug.

According to the *Milbank* report, "distribution was banned by the secretary of Health and Human Services and the pamphlets remained in a warehouse, largely because of strong lobbying and threatened lawsuits by an aspirin-industry-financed organization of pediatricians, the Committee on the Care of Children (CCC), which was created to counteract the warning campaign."

It wasn't until two more years had gone by — and more children had died of RS — that the Department of Health and Human Services (DHHS) finally took the first tentative step to save the lives of other children.

In 1985, DHHS asked the aspirin companies to voluntarily include a warning on aspirin labels, advising people that giving the drug to children with chicken pox or the flu could result in Reye's Syndrome.

It didn't take long to realize that the aspirin companies weren't about to issue any warnings. Finally, in 1986, the government forced them to print aspirin labels with the statement, "Warning: Children and teenagers should not use this medication for chicken pox or flu symptoms before a doctor is consulted about Reye's Syndrome, a rare but serious illness."

The warning was accompanied by a massive public education effort and by 1988 just 20 cases were reported.

A decade later many parents and even some medical doctors have forgotten about the condition.

"In the absence of future controversies about the link between aspirin use and RS...it will be interesting to observe whether the new behaviors will continue," commented the *Milbank* report.

Should those "new behaviors" requiring caution in the giving of aspirin fail to continue, American children may once again find themselves in the middle of a tragic nightmare.

SOURCES:"No aspirin, please," by Gail K. Kaitschuck, *Current Health,* Dec. 1992.

"Effects of professional and media warnings about the association between aspirin use in children and Reye's Syndrome," by Stephen B. Soumerai, Dennis Ross-Degnan, and Jessica Spira Kahn, *The Milbank Quarterly,* Spring 1992.

"Reye's Syndrome surveillance — United States, 1989." *The Journal of the American Medical Association (JAMA),* Feb. 28, 1991.

FDA tries to downplay cancer risk from Ritalin

When the drug methylphenidate (more commonly known by the brand name "Ritalin") was first introduced 40 years ago, drugs makers were not required to test to see whether their product could cause cancer.

In 1995, as part of its routine testing of older drugs, the National Toxicology Program — a branch of the National Institutes of Health — got around to testing Ritalin. It was found that prolonged administration of high doses of the drug administered to mice caused up to four times the expected incidence of cancerous liver tumors.

When advised that Ritalin might cause cancer in mice, the Food & Drug Administration (FDA) merely shrugged. "We felt physicians and parents should know this and have a right to know this. But it's not enough of a signal that we think kids should be taken off the drug," the agency said.

The FDA's only action was to require Ritalin manufacturer Ciba-Geigy Corp., to add the study's findings to the drug's label and notify doctors of the potential risk. The company sent a form letter to 100,000 doctors.

The additional information will be added to the already lengthy description of possible negative side effects associated with the drug.

Even without the new potential for cancer, the drug is considered by many to be unsafe and unnecessary. A listing for Ritalin in the 42nd edition of the "Physicians' Reference," is filled with warnings.

"Sufficient data on safety and efficacy of long-term use of Ritalin in children are not yet available," the book states. "Although a causal relationship has not been established, suppression of growth (i.e., weight gain, and/or height) has been reported with the long-term use of stimulants in children. Therefore, patients requiring long-term therapy should be carefully monitored."

Among the many proven and reported adverse reactions the "Physician's Reference" lists for Ritalin are: nervousness and insomnia; skin rash; fever; anorexia; nausea; dizziness; palpitations; headache; drowsiness; blood pressure and pulse changes; tachycardia; angina; cardiac arrhythmia; abdominal pain; weight loss during prolonged therapy; Tourette's syndrome (rare occurrences); Toxic psychosis; leukopenia and/or anemia; and scalp hair loss.

In 1993, some six million prescriptions for Ritalin and generic versions of the drug were filled, often for children as a "treatment" for hyperactivity.

SOURCES: "Toxicology and Carcinogenesis Studies of Methylphenidate Hydrochloride (CAS No. 298-59-9) in F344/N Rats and B6C3F1 Mice (feed Studies). National Toxicology Program, National Institutes of Health. Report number TR-439, July 1995.

"Cancer in mice fed Ritalin is no cause for fear, FDA says." The Associated Press. Jan. 13, 1996.

Children's ear infections soar despite medical 'treatment'

In 1990, ear infections — known as otitis media — were the second most common diagnosis among all age groups.

Although an estimated *$3-4 billion* is spent every year for medication and surgery, the medical profession has made absolutely no progress in treating or preventing the problem, which is most often seen in children and can result in hearing loss.

While everyone knew it was a common complaint, it wasn't until details of a research study were released that the American public learned just how much worse the problem has become.

According to a 1997 pediatrics journal report, there was a staggering 44% increase in recurrent ear infections among preschool children between 1981 and 1988!

The study found that in 1988, an estimated 5.9 million preschool children had recurrent ear infections in the United States.

One reason that medical science has failed to find an answer to ear infections is that they have for years been looking for the solution in all the wrong places. In fact, despite numerous warnings about the overuse of antibiotics, many M.D.s still routinely prescribe them for young patients with ear infections.

Not long ago, *Ladies Home Journal* reported: "A child's ear infection offers a classic example of how over-treatment with antibiotics can lead to the development of drug- resistant strains of bacteria. For years, amoxicillin — a penicillin-like antibiotic — was the standard treatment for acute otitis media. However, these infections usually clear, without treatment, in two to three days."

The *Journal* noted, though, that "because amoxicillin has been so overprescribed, some ear infections that in the past might have responded to it no longer do. As a result, doctors are forced to prescribe one after another of stronger — and more expensive — medications. Furthermore, the stronger antibiotics are the broad-spectrum ones, which kill the so-called good bacteria as well as the bad, making children vulnerable to secondary infections."

A study published in the *Canadian Family Physician,* by Thomas Lehnert, M.D., CCFP, said that in the United States, 97.9% of children diagnosed with otitis media were given antibiotics by their doctors.

In his study, "Acute Otitis Media in Children: Role of antibiotic therapy," Dr. Lehnert concluded that there was a "definite need for antibiotics in only five-to-ten percent of acute otitis media cases." In the vast majority of cases, the condition is being over-treated.

Unfortunately, many medical doctors don't stop at pumping unneeded antibiotics into children. The other widely used treatment for otitis media, the surgical insertion of tympanotomy tubes, is no improvement.

In 1988, 670,000 of these surgeries were performed in the United States to reduce the frequency of occurrence of otitis media and the potential for resultant hearing loss.

Yet, one medical study indicated that as many as one quarter of the proposed tympanotomy tube insertions *should not have been performed.*

The study, "The Medical Appropriateness of Tympanotomy Tubes Proposed for Children Younger than 16 Years in the United States," published in the *Journal of the American Medical Association (JAMA), was based on 6,611 cases.*

Researchers said that for another third of the cases, there wasn't enough empirical data or expert opinion to support the likelihood of a superior outcome of the tubes over other medical therapy.

To make things worse, insertion of tympanotomy tubes can be risky. Complications include prolonged discharge from the ear, as well as tearing and permanent scarring of the eardrum, which may be associated with low-grade, long-term hearing loss.

The study published in *JAMA* estimated that **several hundred thousand children may be affected annually.** These children may run the risks associated with surgical insertion of tubes even though there is no demonstrated advantage over less invasive therapies.

After looking at research results, many parents are finally realizing that the medical approach to treating ear infections is not only ineffective but dangerous. In most routine cases, they are choosing instead to bolster the child's immune system through diet, behavior modification and natural health care. They are finding that following that strategy allows their children's bodies to ward off infection without the dangers of invasive procedures or drugs.

SOURCES: Pediatrics electronic pages (the Internet extension of *Pediatrics,* the *Journal of the American Academy of Pediatrics,* Feb. 24, 1997.

"A spoonful of medicine: Unnecessary drugs are not only useless, they have the potential to seriously harm our children," by Margery D. Rosen. *Ladies Home Journal,* April 1995 v112 n4 p122(5).

"The medical appropriateness of tympanotomy tubes proposed for children younger than 16 years in the United States. *The Journal of the American Medical Association (JAMA),* April 27, 1994.

Canadian Family Physician, by Thomas Lehnert, M.D., CCFP, "Acute Otitis Media in Children: Role of antibiotic therapy."

Antibiotics should be avoided for middle ear infections

Otitis media is a common childhood ear infection which affects millions of children in the United States and around the world.

For years, nearly all of these children have been given antibiotics for the condition. Some are still infants when doctors pump them full of the drug. In fact, a 1997 medical study showed that 70% of all infants in the U.S. are subjected to their first course of antibiotics before they're even six months old — with otitis media the most common reason for antibiotic treatment.

More evidence has been published to show that antibiotics not only can pose dangers, but they are not effective in treating the problem.

Researchers studied the findings of seven trials comparing antibiotic therapy with placebos in otitis media, and found little evidence to suggest that children given antibiotics had a shorter duration of symptoms, fewer recurrences, or better long term outcomes than those who had received a placebo.

The overuse of antibiotic — such as has happened with children suffering from otitis media — has given rise to a breed of super bacteria which are resistant to antibiotics entirely.

Now, there's even evidence that one of these "superbacteria" — the penicillin-resistant Streptococcus pneumoniae (PRSP) — is actually one of the things that's *causing* otitis media in young children.

This finding was made by Patrick J. Fitzgerald, M.D., of Stanford University, and Joseph B. Robertson, Jr., M.D., and Christina Laane, M.S., of Palo Alto, California.

The results of the research were presented at the 101st Annual Meeting of the American Academy of Otolaryngology — Head and Neck Surgery Foundation, which was held at the Moscone Center in San Francisco, September 7-10, 1997. The meeting was the largest gathering for otolaryngologists (physicians who specialize in the medical and surgical treatment of the ears, nose, throat and related structures of the head and neck).

However, since an estimated *$3-4 billion* is spent every year for medication and surgery to treat the problem, it is unlikely that the medical and drug industries will support either preventive measures or alternative care possibilities.

SOURCES: "Antimicrobials for acute otitis media: A review from the International Primary Care Network," *British Medical Journal*, July 5, 1997.

"Penicillin-Resistant Streptococcus Pneumoniae found in chronic otitis media with effusion," American Academy of Otolaryngology, Sept. 2, 1997.

Asthma treatments called expensive failure

Although billions of dollars have been spent over many years on drug research and related medical treatment of asthma, most of it has been wasted. That was the conclusion of Japanese researcher, Dr. Kazuhiko Kondo.

"Despite widespread use of antiasthmatic drugs," he stated, "the mortality and morbidity due to asthma is increasing worldwide, suggesting the lack of really effective drugs for therapy."

SOURCE: *Journal of Medicinal Chemistry*, published by the American Chemical Society, July 5, 1996.

Allergy shots not helpful for many children with asthma and allergy

Johns Hopkins researchers resolved a longstanding controversy by showing that allergy shots offer little or no benefit to children with year-round, moderate-to-severe asthma.

A 10-year study of 121 children ages five to fourteen with allergies and asthma, showed that the shots had no significant benefits.

"Allergy shots are probably not useful for these patients," said Franklin Adkinson, M.D., a professor of medicine at Hopkins' Asthma and Allergy Center. "This could be because anti-asthma drugs overshadow the shots' effects. It's also possible that exposure to allergens is less important to the start of an asthma episode in these children than we thought."

Patients in the study — funded by the National Institute of Allergy and Infectious Diseases — were sensitive to several airborne allergens, including dust mites, ragweed, grass, oak, and mold. Half were randomly selected to get allergy shots while the other half received inert injections. Patients and their families kept diaries of symptoms and drug use. The study's results were based on that information and on lung function tests.

SOURCE: Media advisory, Johns Hopkins Medical Institutions, Office Of Communications and Public Affairs. January 29, 1997.

Parents get warning about common asthma treatment

According to a report by The Food and Drug Administration (FDA), the popular asthma medication zafirlukast (sold under the name "Accolate"), has been associated with a rare and sometimes fatal condition known as Churg-Strauss Syndrome.

The drug's manufacturer, Zeneca Pharmaceuticals, is now notifying health care providers of this possible drug side effect after the FDA learned of six asthma patients who developed Churg-Strauss Syndrome while taking the drug.

Churg-Strauss Syndrome occurs in adult asthma patients and may appear as generalized, flu- like symptoms such as fever, muscle aches and pains, and weight loss. Patients also experience inflammation of blood vessels, primarily in the lungs. If left untreated, Churg- Strauss Syndrome can result in major organ damage and even death.

Despite the severity of Churg-Strauss Syndrome, the FDA had no plans to prohibit use of zafirlukast/Accolate and told patients not to discontinue its use without consulting their doctor — who prescribed it in the first place.

SOURCE: "Health advisory for new asthma drug," FDA, July 23, 1997.

Shortness being treated as 'disease'

In our society, being tall and thin is the ideal and even children are being pressured to conform to this sometimes unrealistic standard of physical perfection.

Although health officials have often pointed out the damage such pressure can do, an article in *The Journal of the American Medical Association (JAMA)* revealed how dangerous the situation has become.

According to the article, thousands of children who do not suffer from a true growth hormone deficiency are nevertheless being subjected to potentially risky growth hormone therapy — just because they are shorter than average!

Leona Cuttler, M.D., from the Departments of Pediatrics and Pharmacology, School of Medicine, Case Western University, Cleveland, Ohio, and colleagues analyzed the results of a national mail survey of 434 pediatric endocrinologists to determine current opinion and recommendations regarding the controversial issue of growth hormone (GH) use to treat short children.

They found that approximately 58% of current patients undergoing GH therapy have classical GH deficiency, while 42% have other conditions which resulted in their being shorter than average.

The Food and Drug Administration (FDA) has approved growth hormone therapy solely for growth hormone deficiency and chronic renal failure.

The authors explained that the widespread use of GH therapy is due in part to "cultural perceptions about stature." Since being tall is equated with beauty or strength, doctors are often influenced by the child's parents to use GH to increase height — even though there is no true hormone deficiency.

The researchers worried about the risks involved in such therapy, noting that the effect of GH on adult height is not yet known, and the frequency of adverse effects is uncertain.

The authors also brought up another possible reason for the overuse of GH: profit.

"If GH is restricted to children with classical GHD, approximately 14,000 U.S. children are eligible for treatment; this corresponds to an annual cost of approximately $182 million... If non-GHD children with heights below the third percentile are eligible for GH, the pool of candidates increases to 1.7 million children, at an annual cost of $22 billion."

In an accompanying editorial, Barry B. Bercu, M.D., from the University of South Florida, College of Medicine, St. Petersburg, added, "Thought must be given to the idea that GH treatment places children in the role of being sick. Also, the potential psychological damage to the child with unrealistic expectations of what final height will be achieved should also be considered."

As Dr. Bercu explained, "Parental pressure to mitigate short stature in their children is driven by a cultural 'heightism' that permeates American society. Taller college graduates make more money," he continued, "and 80 percent of U.S. presidents have been the taller candidate ...

"Unfortunately there are no definitive long-term controlled studies describing psychological outcome," he pointed out. "There are, however, several psychological studies indicating that short stature per se does not result in negative psychological adaptation.

"One must ask," Bercu concluded, "whether a three-to five-centimeters improvement in height is an acceptable outcome of intervention; it would appear to be less expensive to provide further education, job training, or professional psychological counseling."

SOURCES: "Short stature and growth hormone therapy: a national study of physician recommendation patterns," *The Journal of the American Medical Association (JAMA),* August 21, 1996 v276 n7 p531(7).

"The growing conundrum: growth hormone treatment of the non-growth hormone deficient child." Editorial, *The Journal of the American Medical Association (JAMA)*, August 21, 1996 v276 n7 p567(2).

"Many children treated with growth hormones for social reasons," The American Medical Association, August 20, 1996.

Acne drugs cause serious side effects

One of the most commonly used acne treatments, *minocycline hydrochloride,* produces a blue discoloration of bones in the mouth, reports Dr. Drore Eisen of Dermatology Research Associates, in the British medical journal, *The Lancet.*

Between 1993 and 1996, Eisen examined the mouths of 331 patients who had taken high-dose minocycline for at least six months.

After one year, 33 (10%) of the patients had developed blue bone-discoloration and the proportion increased to 20% after four years. This blue color is permanent in most patients, and in some can be seen through the gums when the patient smiles.

This "blue smile" syndrome is just the latest of numerous reports of serious side effects from the popular acne treatment. In fact, for years medical researchers have suggested possible links between minocycline and liver disease, hepatitis, lupus, and incidents of auto-immune disease.

"Reactions can be severe, so their recognition at an early stage may be important not only to aid recovery but also to avoid invasive investigations such as liver biopsy," researchers stated in the *British Medical Journal.*

"In view of the severity of some reactions, including two deaths and one liver transplant, the use of minocycline for acne should be considered carefully," they added.

Despite these and similar warnings — as well as dire predictions about the dangers of over- prescribing antibiotics in general — many medical doctors still routinely prescribe the antibiotic to their young patients.

SOURCES: "Minocycline induced autoimmune hepatitis and systemic lupus erythematosus-like syndrome." *British Medical Journal,* Jan. 20, 1996.

"Minocycline-induced Autoimmune Disease," *Medical Science Bulletin,* April 1996.

"Acne sufferers to sue firm over 'debilitating' drug." *The (London) Sunday Times,* August 11, 1996.

"Minocycline induced arthritis associated with fever..." *Annals of the Rheumatic Diseases,* Oct. 1996.

The Lancet, February 8, 1997.

Chapter 7

The house of death

Hospitals are supposed to be places where sick people can go to get well. Instead, all too often, they are places where sick people get worse and very sick people die in pain and despair. They're also places which make hundreds of millions of dollars for medical and pharmaceutical companies.

Although there are individuals working in hospitals who are at least well-meaning (if misguided), the main purpose of most hospitals today is to be a profit center for huge health care conglomerates. Administrative and medical decisions are frequently made on the basis of economic advantage, with little attention paid to the needs of the patients or their families.

Worse yet is the fact that many hospitals, particularly those in rural areas, have become the repository of medical personnel who were unable to sustain private practices. Death rates at some of these hospitals have been so high that they have spurred government investigations.

Yet, we flock to hospitals in record number, thinking that we'll find humane and proper health care. We should, instead, heed the advice of most health care advocates: stay out of the hospital at all costs!

Drug side effects in hospitals prolong stay, double risk of death

When a doctor prescribes the wrong drug and a hospitalized person gets worse or dies, hospital administrators don't call it bad medicine — they call it an "adverse drug event," or ADE.

And, although the key promise in the medical Hippocratic Oath is "First, do no harm," ADEs have long been a problem in American hospitals. Three separate research studies published in 1997 revealed just how serious a problem they really are — and the facts shocked health care advocates around the nation.

In the first research report, researchers from LDS Hospital in Salt Lake City, found that ADEs, on average, prolong hospitalizations by nearly two days, cost $2,262 each to treat, and — most frightening of all — almost double the risk of death for patients.

"For several years investigators have studied the prevalence of adverse drug events and found they are a frequent problem. However, this is the first and largest study to examine and quantify the negative ramifications of these drug-related interactions," said David C. Classen, M.D., M.S., lead author of the study and a physician in the department of clinical epidemiology at LDS Hospital.

One of the primary causes of ADEs are the improper interaction between medications, a situation which frequently arises since many patients receive up to 40 different drugs during hospitalization, the report noted.

The LDS Hospital study found that 50% of adverse drug events are preventable.

"The reason that surveillance and intervention programs are absolutely essential is because up to half of all adverse drug events are preventable," said Dr. Classen. "If each event costs an additional $2,262 to treat, as our study shows, and an estimated 30% of all hospitalized patients in the United States experience a drug-reaction, then we are looking at significant opportunity to improve health care and curb unnecessary costs."

Classen pointed out that drug-related morbidity and mortality costs the U.S. more than $86 billion each year. "That's more than the total cost of cardiovascular care or diabetes care in the country," he added.

He also noted that nearly all (92%) of the drug reactions experienced by patients in the study were serious enough to require a change in care as a result of the event.

In a second article, David W. Bates, M.D., M.Sc., from the Division of General Medicine, Brigham and Women's Hospital, Boston, Mass., and colleagues took a closer look at the monetary costs associated with ADEs.

The authors concluded, "We estimated that the annual additional costs associated with preventable ADEs occurring in a large tertiary care hospital were $2.8 million and that the costs associated with all ADEs were $5.6 million. Moreover, these estimates do not include costs of injuries to patients, malpractice costs, or the costs of less serious medication errors or admissions related to ADEs."

Interestingly, it was the high cost in dollars that might prove to be the real incentive for hospitals to decrease these unnecessary — and at times tragic — mistakes.

The study included 4,108 admissions to two hospitals over a six-month period. A self-report by nurses and pharmacists and by daily chart review showed 190 ADEs, of which 60 were preventable. The additional length of stay associated with an ADE was 2.2 days, and the increase in cost associated with an ADE was $3,244. For preventable ADEs, the increases were 4.6 days in length of stay and $5,857 in total cost.

In a third study, conducted by Timothy S. Lesar, Pharm.D., from the Department of Pharmacy, Albany Medical Center, N.Y., and colleagues, the overall error rate was 3.99 per 1,000 medication orders.

The authors found: "Factors commonly associated with errors in prescribing medications were inadequate knowledge or use of knowledge regarding drug therapy; presence of important patient factors related to drug therapy such as age, impaired renal function, and drug allergy; the need for calculation of drug doses; and specialized dosage formulation characteristics and medication prescribing nomenclature."

The study indicated that about 12% of the mistakes involved giving patients drugs to which they were allergic; 11% involved giving the wrong drug; and 11% involved prescribing the wrong dosage.

In an editorial for the *Journal of the American Medical Association,* which published the three papers, Jerry Avorn, M.D., from the Program for the Analysis of Clinical Strategies, Brigham and Women's Hospital, Harvard Medical School, Boston, Mass., stated the studies clearly showed that "ADEs in hospitalized patients are countable, dangerous, and evaluable events, not just a collection of unhappy accidents that strike, like cosmic rays, in ways that we cannot predict or understand."

He called on hospitals to crack down on the frequency of ADEs. "These articles make a good case for the need to pay far more attention to these important causes of morbidity, mortality, and resource use," he noted. "Whatever the precise measure of their impact, their toll in human and fiscal terms is clearly large enough to justify commitment of hospital resources to programs designed to reduce preventable ADEs to the lowest possible incidence."

SOURCES: "LDS Hospital Study finds that adverse drug events cost thousands to treat, prolong hospitalizations by two days, and nearly double risk of death," by LDS Hospital, Salt Lake City, Jan. 21, 1997.

"Drug Errors Costly to Health Care System," American Medical Association, Jan. 22, 1997.

"Reducing Hospital Medication Prescribing Errors," Albany Medical Center, Jan. 18, 1997.

The Journal of the American Medical Association, Jan. 22, 1997.

Math errors lead to hospital tragedies

News of the increasing number of medical errors which injure or kill patients — particularly in hospitals — is shocking. But usually, the studies conducted on this serious problem contain pages and pages of statistics, providing little insight into the human suffering behind the figures.

In London not long ago, medical tragedy was given a very real face — that of a premature baby who died within an hour of being given a hundred times the intended dose of morphine.

The coroner at the inquest commented that doctors should not be allowed to practice until they showed a "tolerable ability" in mathematics.

That newborn baby is just one sad example of medical incompetence and mistakes, often caused by sloppy writing of figures in prescriptions and drug orders.

The medical communities in the U.S. and around the world have tried to decrease the problem by instructing medical personnel to print instructions neatly, avoid using decimal points whenever possible, or put a "zero" before the decimal point when appropriate.

Those recommendations, however, assume the tragedies stem from misinterpretation of handwritten notes. Obviously, that's not the only cause of medical errors involving wrong drug dosages.

All too often, the mistakes are a result of carelessness and what the editor of *The Lancet* has called "a momentary mental block — the kind of block that causes a person to make simple errors such as dividing rather than multiplying by a conversion factor or vice versa."

Compounding the problem is the fact that nurses — the people who used to double check doctors' drug orders and frequently catch mistakes before they became tragedies — are no longer effective 'fail safe' mechanisms.

In fact, in some areas of the U.S., complaints about nurses have as much as tripled in the past few years. In Massachusetts, for instance, there has been a backlog of as many as 600 complaint cases filed against nurses.

"The workload has increased, the patients are sicker and we are doing more things with more responsibility than ever before," explained one nurse administrator.

Since Massachusetts has only three investigators to oversee its 120,000 licensed nurses, ensuring their competency has become nearly impossible.

In one case, a nurse was able to renew her Massachusetts nursing license even though she was a drug addict with drug convictions and a revoked California license.

According to a report in *American Medical News:* "It took four years for the state to revoke the license of a nurse who was stealing painkillers from a hospital. She continued to work even after her license was revoked."

SOURCES: American Medical News, November 11, 1996.
The Lancet February 8, 1997.

Hospital-caused infections on the rise

When patients are admitted into hospitals, one of the biggest health problems they face isn't necessarily the one they went in with. They must battle infections they are likely to acquire during their stay.

Now there is an added danger.

Bacterial infections resistant to a potent antibiotic are increasing in hospitals and are associated with a high death rate, according to infectious disease researchers at Northwestern University Medical School.

A bacteria with growing resistance to the broad-spectrum antibiotic vancomycin — enterococcus faecium — has been implicated as a major cause of hospital-acquired infections.

In a study of 53 patients with enterococcal infections, Valentina Stosor, M.D., and colleagues found that **all 21 cases of vancomycin-resistant infec-**

tions were acquired in the hospital. All of the patients had received treatment with vancomycin previously.

Of this group, 75% of the patients died — most from complications of the infection.

Twenty five of the other 32 cases — which were not resistant to vancomycin — also acquired the infection in the hospital. In this group, 40% died from their illness.

All patients had received a variety of broad-spectrum antibiotics before developing the bacteria in their blood, possibly weakening their immune systems and making them more vulnerable to the infection.

In addition to a higher mortality rate, the resistant infections cost on average about $25,000 more to treat and doubled the patients' length of stay in the hospital.

According to Gary A. Noskin, M.D., assistant professor of medicine and one of the researchers on the Northwestern study, these results raise important issues regarding overuse of antibiotics by physicians among hospitalized patients.

"Antibiotic-resistant bacteria have emerged as a serious problem among hospitalized patients. In addition to the high mortality associated with these infections, they are very costly to treat," Noskin said.

SOURCE: "Hospital Acquired Infections," Northwestern University, Sept. 11, 1996.

U.S. for-profit hospitals overspend on red tape

Medical supporters often try to justify the soaring costs of hospital stays by saying the fees are used for better medical care. However, according to Harvard Medical School researcher Steffie Woolhandler and Sidney Wolfe of Public Citizen's Health Research Group, that money is more likely to go for increased administrative costs.

In a report published in *The New England Journal of Medicine,* the researchers concluded that U.S. for-profit hospitals are diverting money from patient care and using it instead for administrative expenses.

Not only did the study show that the hospitals are increasingly putting their own business needs before the health needs of patients, it also noted that overall costs are higher at for-profits than at private non-profit or public facilities, which Wolfe said "unearths the fallacy of efficiency" of for-profits.

Spending on clinical personnel for each hospital stay in 1994 was $2,954 at for-profits, $3,296 at non-profits, and $2,909 at public hospitals, according to the study. Overall costs per stay were higher at for-profits, largely due to administrative costs, said the authors.

SOURCE: "Costs of care and administration at for-profit and other hospitals in the United States," *The New England Journal of Medicine (NEJM),* March 13, 1997.

Hospital neglect causes spread of TB

Two outbreaks of tuberculosis have been linked to contaminated hospital bronchoscopes, according to two separate articles in the October 1, 1997 issue of *The Journal of the American Medical Association (JAMA).*

Tracy Agerton, R.N., M.P.H., from the Centers for Disease Control and Prevention in Atlanta, and colleagues studied the spread in South Carolina of a rare strain of Mycobacterium tuberculosis (TB) that is resistant to seven first-line anti-tuberculosis medications.

In a separate article, Theresa M. Michele, M.D., of Johns Hopkins University School of Medicine in Baltimore, and colleagues provided evidence that TB was transmitted from one person to another via a contaminated bronchoscope at an unidentified hospital.

Bronchoscopes are instruments used to examine the lung's airways. Bronchoscopies occasionally are performed to confirm the diagnosis of TB, which is usually passed in airborne droplets produced by coughing or sneezing.

The researchers were able to link the spread of TB through dirty bronchoscopes by using DNA fingerprinting and extensive epidemiological investigations.

Both studies found that hospitals failed to adequately clean and disinfect used bronchoscopes, according to nationally established guidelines. TB was spread from one infected patient to other patients who subsequently underwent bronchoscopies with the same instrument.

Agerton and colleagues found that five of the eight people with a rare, drug-resistant strain of TB in South Carolina in early 1995 were family members or a close friend, confirming close contact and normal transmittal by air. However, three additional people who contracted the same strain of TB with "identical" DNA fingerprints had no contact with the others except for a hospital bronchoscope.

Both studies said the hospitals did not adequately clean and disinfect used bronchoscopes, according to guidelines established by the Association for Practitioners in Infection Control. Both studies suggested following more vigilant cleaning techniques called for by some manufacturers and the Food and Drug Administration.

SOURCE: "Contaminated bronchoscopes spread TB," *The Journal of the American Medical Association (JAMA),* Oct. 1, 1997.

Hospitals slapped with fine in playwright's death

After working for 10 years as a waiter, living in a lower Manhattan tenement, 35-year-old Jonathan Larson was finally on the verge of success as a playwright. His play, "Rent," was about to open off-Broadway and — though he didn't know it at the time — it would be such a phenomenal triumph that it would not only move to Broadway on April 29, 1996, but would go on to win four Tonys and a Pulitzer Prize for drama.

But Larson never got to enjoy the success he worked so hard for. He never heard the cheers of the Broadway audiences or read the rave reviews in the

New York papers. He never got to hold his awards or look forward to writing another play.

Larson died in January after doctors at two different hospital emergency rooms failed to correctly diagnose the aneurysm that killed him. Although he complained of severe chest pains, ER doctors at one hospital told him he was suffering from food poisoning. Doctors at the other said it was a virus. Both hospitals sent him home, where he died.

After its four-month investigation showed that the hospitals did misdiagnose the problem, the New York Health Department fined them a mere $16,000 and shrugged the tragedy off by explaining that a correct diagnosis "would have been extremely difficult," since he wasn't in a high risk group for the type of aneurysm he had.

SOURCE: American Medical News, Jan. 13, 1997.

Study finds hospital patients lack vital information at discharge

Many physicians overestimate how much their patients understand about treatment following a hospital stay, according to David R. Calkins, M.D., of the University of Kansas School of Medicine in Kansas City, and his colleagues.

The researchers surveyed 99 patients and their attending physicians. All of the patients were treated at Beth Israel Hospital in Boston between October, 1991 and December, 1992. All were treated for either pneumonia or acute myocardial infarction (heart attack). Both conditions have significant post-discharge treatment requirements.

In the survey, the researchers asked both the doctors and the patients various questions, including how long the doctor spent talking to them about their care needs once they left the hospital, and how much the patients actually understood of the discussion.

They found that doctors reported spending more time talking about post-discharge care than patients did. In almost half the cases (43.1%), the patient thought less time had been spent than the physician reported.

Although there was not way to determine how much time doctors *actually* spent talking to their patients, it was obvious that the perception between patient and professional differed greatly.

In fact, the researchers found, "Patients and physicians agreed about the amount of time spent discussing post-discharge care only 32.3% of the time."

Patients and doctors also differed on how much the patients understood about the side effects of medication the patients would be taking after leaving the hospital.

"Physicians believed that 88.9% of patients understood potential side effects of post-discharge medication, but only 57.4% of patients reported that they understood," the researchers wrote.

The researchers also asked physicians and patients about the resumption of normal activities following hospitalization. They found: "Physicians believed that 94.7% of patients knew when to resume normal activities, whereas only 57.9% of patients reported that they knew when normal activities could resume."

The researchers conclusion: "Inadequate preparation for discharge and non-compliance with treatment plans following discharge have been associated with an increased risk of unplanned readmission. It is certainly possible that better understanding of the side effects of medications and of the appropriate time to resume normal activities would reduce the risk of unplanned readmission or improve other outcomes of care following hospital discharge."

SOURCE: The Archives of Internal Medicine, May 12, 1997.

Research finds that hospital food flunks nutrition tests

Medical doctors have often been criticized for their ignorance about nutrition — their education includes *almost no training* on this important health topic. Now, however, it's been discovered that university teaching hospitals apparently don't know the basics about nutrition either.

In fact, a computerized analysis of the nutritional value of the house diets offered in 57 university teaching hospitals showed that only *four* met all seven of the recommendations of the National Research Council (NRC).

Measurement was made of content in four component areas: fat, saturated fat, cholesterol and sodium. Results revealed that 22 (39%) of the hospitals exceeded the acceptable target for fat content, 27 (47%) saturated fat, 46 (81%) cholesterol, and 31 (54%) failed to keep within safe limits of sodium content in the food.

Twelve percent of the hospitals analyzed offered menus which did not provide an adequate number of servings of fruits and vegetables. Fewer than half (44%) provided patients with any information concerning the nutritional value of dietary items.

The medical doctors who performed the survey concluded that "many teaching hospitals do not design house diets to meet nationally recognized dietary recommendations and do not supply patients with enough information to help them make healthful dietary choices. These discouraging results are consistent with those of a report by Israeli investigators, who found that none of that country's university hospitals served diets that met the dietary goals of the American Heart Association."

They recommended that, "Hospitals should assume a greater role in promoting more healthful diets. We cannot think of a more appropriate place to encourage the nutritional health of Americans."

SOURCE: New England Journal of Medicine, November 7, 1996.

Chapter 8

The vaccine myth

What conquered polio?

If you're like most Americans, you probably believe it was a vaccine which rescued the human race from this tragic illness. But there is mounting evidence that the terrible polio epidemic of the 1930s and '40s was a normal, temporary episode of the disease which was already running its course when the polio vaccine was developed. The disease petered out around the world at about the same time — even in countries which did not employ the vaccine. Similar epidemics have come, and gone, throughout history.

The perception, however, that the vaccine was responsible for the decline of polio caused the medical profession to rush into the vaccine industry, creating drugs which were supposedly capable of "improving" the body's immune system to ward off diseases.

In fact, however, those vaccines are now threatening the very immune systems they are suppose to support. Every year, medical studies are sounding warning alarms that we may be causing irreparable damage to the human system — especially in children — through unnecessary and potentially harmful vaccines.

But those alarms are being drowned out by the pro-vaccine campaigns which are funded almost entirely by drug companies which make billions of dollars producing and selling the vaccines.

Their efforts to hide the truth about the dangers of vaccines have been so successful that few parents in America are even aware that the government was forced to set up a special "compensation" fund to reimburse the families of children who were killed or injured as a result of mandatory vaccines. Instead, the public is told only that their children's health depends on these drugs.

How long will we continue to believe the lies?

Group warns against new chicken pox vaccine

The National Vaccine Information Center (NVIC) is continuing its efforts to make the chicken pox vaccine voluntary rather than mandatory.

The group warns that the government's recommendation to inject all *healthy* children with the new live virus vaccine may cause more serious disease when they become adults.

A mild disease for most children, chicken pox is caused by the varicella zoster virus, a relative of the herpes virus. A vaccine was originally developed to protect high-risk individuals — particularly children with leukemia, kidney disease or immune suppression, etc. — from serious complications such as brain damage and death.

However, the Centers for Disease Control (CDC) and the American Academy of Pediatrics (AAP) have recommended that **ALL** children 12-15 months old and individuals over age 13 who have not had chicken pox, be injected with a vaccine developed by Merck & Co.

"The question is: 'Is what is good for all *high-risk* children also good for all healthy children?,'" said Barbara Loe Fisher, NVIC president. "When you recover from the natural disease, which is very mild in most children, you are usually immune for life. We know this vaccine only gives temporary immunity — perhaps five-to-ten years' worth. There is a real danger that if everyone gets vaccinated, chicken pox will become an adult disease where it can be much more deadly.

"At the same time," she continued, "no one knows if the live vaccine virus will lay dormant in many vaccinated individuals and reactivate later in life in the form of herpes zoster (shingles) or other immune system disorders."

The death rate for chicken pox is 1.4 per 100,000 cases in healthy children but rises to nearly 31 per 100,000 cases in adults. According to the U.S. government, chicken pox results in more than 9,000 hospitalizations annually and causes between 50 and 100 deaths — mostly in adults.

A 1994 CDC study estimated $439 million per year is spent by parents in time lost from work caring for children with chicken pox. One of the primary justifications for recommendations that all children be vaccinated has been to spare parents from having to miss work time.

"Chicken pox is not smallpox," Fisher pointed out. "The benefit risk ratio for healthy children is much different than for high risk children. The chicken pox vaccine should not be mandated. Parents should be able to choose whether or not they want their children to be vaccinated and get a temporary immunity, which will probably require booster vaccinations throughout life, or have the natural disease and get permanent immunity for life."

Continuing questions about efficacy and long-term side effects stalled the licensure of a chicken pox vaccine in America for several years. The FDA estimates the chicken pox vaccine is about 70-90% effective in preventing the disease. Common short-term side effects include redness, hardness and swelling at the injection site, as well as fatigue and nausea. Long-term side effects are unknown because children in the studies used to license the vaccine were only followed up for 10 years. The live virus vaccine will cost physicians $39 per dose.

SOURCE: Special Report from The National Vaccine Information Center (NVIC).

Major HMO gave 'thumbs down' to chickenpox vaccine

A major west coast Health Maintenance Organization (HMO) announced in 1996 that, based on mounting criticism from health agencies and leading pediatricians, it would not recommend the chickenpox vaccine to its patients.

Pacificare Health Systems stated that it was concerned that the vaccine would wear off years after it is administered, leaving adults vulnerable to the disease at a time when it can be much more serious.

For the vast majority of children, chickenpox is a mild childhood disease and provides the child with a natural, lifetime immunity. The long-term effectiveness of the medically developed vaccine, manufactured under the name "Varivax," is uncertain and some experts are unconvinced that any protection it affords will last past adolescence.

If the vaccine "wears off," people would then be vulnerable to the disease which can pose far more serious risks to adults. Although some critics accused the HMO of rejecting the vaccine because of its costs, Dr. William Osheroff, medical director of Pacificare's California HMOs stressed that, "The real issue is all of the unanswered questions about Varivax, not cost." He added that the HMO would offer the vaccine to parents who requested it, but would not endorse or recommend it.

"This is a very benign disease in children, but the vaccine may create a false sense of security as these kids get older and find themselves non-immune," he said. "Chickenpox as an adult is a serious disease."

SOURCE: Associated Press, April 2, 1996.

Vaccine many cause Crohn's disease

According to a research study published in a prestigious British medical journal, there may be a direct link between the measles vaccine and Crohn's disease.

Medical doctors at the Royal Free Hospital of Medicine reported that children who were vaccinated for that common childhood ailment have a significantly higher risk of developing Crohn's disease and ulcerative colitis later in life than non-vaccinated children.

The doctors compared 3,545 people who had received live measles vaccine in 1964 to a control group of 11,407 people. By 1994, three times as many people in the vaccinated group had developed Crohn's disease and twice as many had developed ulcerative colitis when compared to the unvaccinated group.

The study reinforced many researchers' fears that exposure to the measles virus can cause a prolonged disruption in the immune function.

SOURCE: *The Lancet* Vol. 345, April 29, 1995, pp. 1071-74.

Possible link between vaccines and diabetes examined

A study conducted by researchers at InterMountain Health Care's LDS Hospital in Salt Lake City and Classen Immunotherapies in Baltimore, showed that immunization with the BCG vaccine (a common vaccine used to prevent tuberculosis) starting at school age may be associated with a substantially increased risk of insulin-dependent diabetes.

The research also linked rises in the incidence of the disease, also know as Type 1 diabetes, to the administration of the hepatitis B and hemophilus B vaccine in children who were vaccinated after they were two-months old.

The results of the analysis were published the October 22, 1997 issue of the journal, *Infectious Diseases in Clinical Practices.*

The study was released just one week before the Centers for Disease Control and Prevention (CDC) announced that the number of Americans with diabetes was at its highest level ever at 15.7 million diabetics in the U.S. in 1997 or close to six percent of the population.

Incredibly, the medical establishment's response was to suggest that children receive the vaccine **at birth** rather than wait until they are eight weeks old! They claim that this will reduce the risk, although they admit they are not even sure as to why the drugs cause the increase in diabetes.

Lead researcher Dr. David Classen suggested that immunization with a wide variety of vaccines may alter the risk of Type 1 diabetes by the release of interferon and other immune mediators in a newborn's system.

"Interferon released at birth following immunization may prevent children from being colonized with diabetes-inducing viruses from their mother," he said. "By contrast, after children are eight weeks or older they may have subclinical inflammation of insulin secreting cells that may be enhanced by immunization leading to insulin dependent diabetes."

Dr. Classen, however, could not say with certainty that subjecting the newborns with the drugs would actually prevent diabetes or if it might cause other, possibly more serious health problems.

One thing he was definite about: More than $30 billion is spent annually in the U.S. alone to treat people with insulin-dependent diabetes.

SOURCES: "Childhood Diabetes May Be Linked To Immunizations," InterMountain Health Care, Oct. 24, 1997.

U.S. Department of Health and Human Services, Centers for Disease Control Press Release, Oct. 30, 1997.

Flu deaths up despite "vaccine"

Every year, government agencies and medical doctors stress the need for people to get their annual flu shots. Although they started out recommending it only for people in high risk groups such as the elderly, many doctors are now urging everyone — even young, healthy adults — to get the influenza vaccine.

Although the vaccine is supposed to protect them from the ravishes of the flu, which for most people is — at worst — a short-lived inconvenience, it appears that the flu shot may be less effective than even the most pessimistic observer could have predicted.

According to figures released in February 1996 by the Centers for Disease

Control, the number of deaths attributed to the flu *increased significantly* in 1993 — with more than 82,820 people dying from the illness.

The number of flu-related deaths was so high that it actually had an impact on average life expectancy figures. Flu and pneumonia are the sixth leading cause of death despite the widespread use of vaccines, which carry their own risks of negative side effects.

SOURCES: Centers for Disease Control, Feb. 29, 1996.

The Associated Press, "Flu deaths spur drop in life expectancy," March 1, 1996.

Immunizations can cause hair loss

Routine immunization may be the trigger for cases of unexpected hair loss, according to an article in the October 8, 1997 issue of *The Journal of the American Medical Association (JAMA)*. It stated that the incidence of hair loss is considered rare, even though there have been reported cases on record for nearly 30 years.

Robert P. Wise, M.D., M.P.H., from the Food and Drug Administration (FDA) in Rockville, Md., and colleagues began investigating reports of hair loss following vaccination after receiving a report in 1994 from a concerned mother whose 12-month-old daughter began losing her hair 10 days after receiving a second dose of hepatitis B vaccine.

The researchers discovered cases of hair loss after vaccination dating back to 1969. For this study, they evaluated 60 reports of hair loss submitted since 1984.

They found:
➤ Patients' ages varied from two months to 67 years.
➤ The majority of cases were among women (49 of 59 patients for whom sex was reported).
➤ Forty-six of the 60 people had received hepatitis B vaccine.
➤ Sixteen reported hair loss following vaccination on more than one occasion.

The degree and duration of hair loss varied widely.

Of the 37 reports with information sufficient to classify the extent of hair loss, approximately half had extensive hair loss and half had mild-to- moderate hair loss (with most hair still intact). However, the extent of hair re-growth also varied.

SOURCE: The Journal of the American Medical Association (JAMA), October 8, 1997.

Higher-risk polio vaccine called more cost effective

For decades, health care advocates have warned about the possible risks of administering live oral polio vaccines. Instead, they have urged the use of an inactivated vaccine which is less likely to cause polio.

A study by medical researchers gave a clear indication of why the switch has not been made: MONEY.

The U.S. pays more than $11 million each year in settlements with people who contract polio from the oral vaccine. Changing to the less risky type of vaccine would cost $28 million. Apparently, it's cheaper to stick with the live vaccine and sacrifice a certain number of people to lifelong disabilities.

The researchers noted: "The introduction of [inactivated polio vaccine] into the routine vaccination schedule would not be cost-beneficial at current vaccine prices and with the current compensation awards paid to vaccine-associated poliomyelitis cases."

They acknowledged that concern is growing about the safety of the current live vaccine, and stated that the higher expense "may be justified to assuage public concerns about adverse events associated with a government mandated vaccination program."

Unfortunately, the study did not address the ethical question of making potential life-altering decisions based on monetary considerations.

SOURCES: Cost-effectiveness of incorporating inactivated poliovirus vaccine into the routine childhood immunization schedule," Mark A. Miller, Roland W. Sutter, Peter M. Strebel, and Stephen C. Hadler. *The Journal of the American Medical Association (JAMA),* Sept. 25, 1996.

"Inactive polio vaccine may not be cost effective," *American Medical News,* October 7, 1996.

Women suffer side effects from rubella vaccine

Most of the criticism about vaccines center around the harm they can do to children. However, the side effects which one vaccine causes in women have been uncovered.

The rubella (German measles) vaccine has been available since the 1960s and since then, reports have shown that between 10% and 40% of women who previously had no immunity to rubella experience joint disorders that can cause pain in joints such as the ankles and knees after getting the vaccine.

In 1997, Professor Aubrey Tingle and colleagues from Vancouver, British Columbia, Canada, reported on their study of acute and recurrent joint and neurological problems in previously healthy women who received the vaccine shot shortly after giving birth.

All 546 women were vaccinated within three months of giving birth. To compare the rate of adverse events in the joints that could be associated with the vaccine, 270 women were given a rubella vaccine and 276 women were injected with saline solution. The women did not know which kind of shot they received.

Before the women gave birth, they were visited in their homes, at which time a detailed medical history was taken and a rheumatological examination was done to check for previous joint disorders. Four weeks after vaccination, patients were visited in the home again and any joint or muscle pain that they had experienced was recorded by a trained nurse.

Similar reports were taken from patients at 3, 6, 9, and 12 months, when a final physical assessment was made.

The authors found that there were significant differences in the rate of occurrence of acute adverse joint manifestations between the vaccine and placebo groups.

SOURCE: *The Lancet,* May 3, 1997.

'Stealth' virus warning issued

In 1995, the National Vaccine Information Center (NVIC) released a special alert concerning the growing threat of "stealth" viruses which may be invading the U.S. through live viral vaccines.

According to the Center, studies by W. John Martin, M.D., Ph.D., pathologist and immunologist at the University of Southern California, began raising disturbing questions about a class of "atypical cytopathic" viruses — viruses which can cause pathologic changes in human cells.

These viruses — dubbed "stealth" viruses because they are able to invade the body without setting off its normal cellular defense mechanisms — "appear to lack the antigens which normally cause an inflammation typical of most infections that damage cells and body tissues," the Center reported.

The NVIC, which maintains an extensive, worldwide database of information concerning the adverse effects of vaccines, was alerted to the "stealth virus" situation after Dr. Martin had used DNA sequence analysis to identify one of the viruses as being of African green monkey origin. Kidney tissues from these animals were used to make the live oral polio vaccine, as well as other viral vaccines during the past three decades, the Center explained.

Martin, professor of pathology and director of USC's Infectious Diseases and Molecular Pathology Lab, urged the FDA to research the problem and take immediate action to avoid widespread health risks.

"The FDA is responsible for the safety of biological products including vaccines and the nation's blood supply," he told government officials.

While Martin and his colleagues tackled the FDA and sought a research solution, the NVIC continued to expand the scope of its 14-year-old vaccine reaction registry and began collecting information and providing referrals for those suffering from unexplained neurological, psychiatric and autoimmune disorder symptoms that are potentially related to stealth virus infection.

SOURCE:*The Vaccine Reaction,* National Vaccine Information Center. Barbara Loe Fisher, Ed. "Discovery of an atypical virus infecting human linked to viral vaccines produced on money tissues," Sept/Oct 1995. Special report.

Why should hepatitis B vaccine be given to all children?

by Barbara Loe Fisher

Nineteen states have passed laws requiring three doses of hepatitis B vaccine for all healthy children. Most 12-hour-old newborns can't leave the newborn nurseries of hospitals without being injected with hepatitis B virus vaccine.

Why?

Not content with using the hepatitis B vaccine in high risk populations such as IV drug users, prostitutes, prisoners and sexually promiscuous adults for which this vaccine was created, drug companies and officials at the Centers for Disease Control (CDC) have targeted vulnerable newborns in the first moments of life to find a larger and more reliable market for their produce.

Using the justification that babies born to mothers infected with hepatitis B disease have an 85-95% risk of developing chronic hepatitis B infection and promoting the idea that injecting all healthy babies with hepatitis B vaccine will protect them when they are teenagers and become sexually active, CDC officials have convinced state health departments to add hepatitis B vaccine to the list of mandatory vaccinations.

But a quick check of the CDC's own statistics, drug company product inserts and medical texts such as "Harrison's Principles of Internal Medicine" and "The Merck Manual," as well as a 1994 report from the Institute of Medicine, tell a different story from the one promoted in CDC press releases.

Consider the following facts:

1. Hepatitis B is spread by direct contact with infected body fluids such as blood and semen.

Question: How many babies does this apply to?

2. In 1995, there were less than 300 cases of hepatitis B disease reported in the U.S. in children under 14.

Question: Who did the cost-benefit analysis to justify injecting three-and-a-half million newborns with hepatitis B virus to try to prevent 300 cases? A drug company executive?

3. Hepatitis B is most prevalent in the Far East and Africa (10% of the population) with the lowest incidence in the world being in the U.S. and western Europe (0.1% to 0.5%).

Question: So why does EVERY American child need to get vaccinated to solve a problem in the Far East and Africa?

4. Ninety-to-ninety five percent of hepatitis B cases recover completely after three-to-four weeks of nausea, fatigue, headache, cough, arthralgia, jaundice and tender liver and are left with permanent immunity. The case-fatality ratio is low, approximately 0.1% to 1.4%.

Question: Why has the CDC felt it necessary to scare the public into believing hepatitis B virus is deadly enough to justify making every American take the vaccine?

5. In 1994, the Institute of Medicine reported that there is compelling scientific evidence to conclude that hepatitis B vaccine can cause shock that can end in death. Because either no studies or too few studies have ever been conducted to investigate the impact of hepatitis B vaccine on the body, a determination could not be made as to whether or not hepatitis B vaccine causes Guillain-Barre syndrome; central demyelinating diseases of the brain such as transverse myelitis, optic neuritis or multiple sclerosis; acute or chronic arthritis or sudden infant death syndrome (SIDS).

Question: What, precisely, DO public health officials know about this vaccine?

6. The CDC states: "Between 30% to 50% of persons who develop adequate antibody after three doses of vaccine will lose detectable antibody within 7 years."

Question: What was that about vaccinating our newborns to protect them when they get to be teenagers?

7. According to a hepatitis B vaccine manufacturer: "The duration of protective effect [of the vaccine] is unknown at present and the need for booster doses is not yet defined."

Question: How many think this drug company statement is a set-up for a very profitable future one that will recommend booster doses for every American throughout life?

8. Before the hepatitis B vaccine was widely used, in 1989 there were 23,419 cases of hepatitis B disease reported in the U.S. with 711 deaths. In 1994, there were 12,517 cases reported and the CDC stated "Hepatitis B continues to decline in most states primarily because of changes in high-risk behaviors among injecting drug-users."

Case closed.

(Barbara Loe Fisher, co-author of "DPT: A Shot in the Dark" and a co-founder and president of the National Vaccine Information Center, served on the National Vaccine Advisory Committee for four years and is a member of the Vaccine Safety Forum at the Institute of Medicine. She is the editor of a national, bi-monthly newsletter, The Vaccine Reaction, and is on the editorial board of the Journal of Vertebral Subluxation Research. She has appeared on hundreds of radio and television programs, including "The Today Show," "CBS Evening News" and "Nightline," and speaks at health care conferences and town meetings advocating the human right to informed consent to any medical intervention which carries the risk of injury or death, including vaccination.)

SOURCE: Reprinted, with permission, from *The Chiropractic Journal,* May 1997.

Contaminated polio vaccines cause national protests

When the American Academy of Pediatrics (AAP) released polio vaccine recommendations in 1996, the National Vaccine Information Center (NVIC) called it a "step in the right direction."

After all, the recommendations gave parents the right to choose what kind of polio vaccine their children will receive. However, according to NVIC officials, parents wouldn't know what choice to make unless doctors first gave them full and complete information about **all** of the risks of polio vaccines.

In addition, responding to reports in *New York* and *Money* magazines, the vaccine safety advocate group called on vaccine manufacturers to stop using monkeys to produce polio vaccines because of scientific evidence that polio vaccines contaminated with monkey viruses are linked with cancer and other serious health problems in children and adults.

"For 40 years, parents have been kept in the dark by vaccine policy makers and manufacturers about the risks of both live and inactivated polio vaccines," stated NVIC co- founder and president Barbara Loe Fisher. "It is about time that parents are given full information about both kinds of polio vaccines and are allowed to make educated decisions for their children. Part of the information they need to know is that polio vaccines grown on monkey kidney tissues have been found to be contaminated with monkey viruses."

The live oral polio vaccine (OPV), which has been used almost exclusively since the 1960s, can actually give the vaccinated children polio. The disease can also be transmitted to parents, babysitters, or other persons who come into contact with a recently vaccinated child.

Since 1979, the only cases of polio which occurred in American children and adults are caused by OPV. The inactivated polio vaccine (IPV), which was the first kind of polio vaccine to be developed in the 1950s, does not have the ability to cause polio in the vaccinated person or close contacts.

In June 1996, the Centers for Disease Control issued a new recommendation calling for a national polio vaccine policy change to cut down on the number of vaccine-associated polio cases and recommended IPV be used for the first two doses, and OPV be used for the second two doses.

According to the NVIC, the policy reduces — but does not eliminate — the number of vaccine-associated polio cases in the U.S. Families whose members are suffering from vaccine-strain polio have called for an all-IPV schedule to be implemented immediately. This is the step taken by France in 1983, when it made the decision to eliminate all forms of polio, both wild and vaccine-strain, in that country.

On November 11, 1996, *New York* magazine ran an investigative report on the contamination of OPV and IPV with monkey viruses. A similar investigative article was published in the December 1996 issue of *Money* magazine. Both investigations revealed that OPV and IPV are grown on monkey kidney tissues and that scientists in the U.S. and around the world are beginning to identify monkey virus genes and proteins in children and adults with bone, brain and lung cancers, as well as immune and neurological disorders.

"There is evidence that vaccine manufacturers and government regulators knew in the late 1950s and early 1960s that the polio vaccines were contaminated with monkey viruses but chose to continue producing vaccines using monkey tissues rather than develop alternative ways to make both vaccines," stated Fisher.

"All polio vaccines using monkeys for production should be removed from the market until there is a full scientific investigation into the contamination problem," she charged. "There is an inactivated polio vaccine grown on human lung cells that is used in other countries but not in America. Parents should demand that it be made available for American children."

Lederly Laboratories, which makes and sells OPV in the U.S., and Connaught Laboratories, which makes and sells IPV in the U.S., both use African Green monkey kidney cells to make their vaccines. However, Connaught also makes an IPV vaccine grown on human lung cells which it sells in other countries.

SOURCES: The National Vaccine Information Center (512 W. Maple Ave., #206, Vienna, VA 22180), Nov. 14, 1996.

Money Magazine, December 1996.

New York Nov. 11, 1996.

Parents not told that measles vaccine was experimental

A major research project involving two measles vaccines was conducted on 1,500 minority infants in Los Angeles starting in 1989 — and parents were never told that one of the vaccines was experimental.

Dr. David Satcher, the director of the Centers for Disease Control (CDC) — which approved the trial — admitted the government-sponsored experiment put children at risk without proper disclosure, but called it "a little mistake."

Although stating that the CDC considered the matter "serious," he shrugged it off by explaining, "Things sometimes fall through the cracks." The experiment was conducted by Kaiser Permanente, a major vaccine manufacturer.

Although the use of the experimental drug on the L.A. children had not been linked to any health problems when news of this project became known, other children weren't so lucky.

A similar trial conducted in Haiti and Africa *did* come under scrutiny. In that experiment, female infants who received the more powerful of the doses suffered an increased death rate. When knowledge of this effect was learned in 1991, the Los Angeles study was discontinued.

The experimental vaccine used on the California infants was not licensed in the United States.

SOURCE: "Study didn't tell parents trial vaccine was used." *Los Angeles Times* June 16, 1996.

Chapter 9

Wolves guarding the sheep

The American people normally feel safe about drugs they take because they are "approved" by the federal government's Food and Drug Administration (FDA). That may have been true at one time, but the agency has become, in recent years, little more than a business partner to the drug industry.

Changes in FDA rules — like a speeded up approval process — almost always benefit the drug companies. Its double standard in approving dangerous drugs while attacking beneficial vitamin supplements has become so obvious that even its most ardent supporters have trouble justifying its actions.

FDA applies double standard in policing "dangerous" drugs

In April 1996, the Food & Drug Administration (FDA) announced that a prescription pain reliever it approved the previous year was linked to more than 80 cases of seizures. It also admitted getting 115 reports of drug abuse, dependence, withdrawal or intentional overdose by its users.

Yet, its only actions were to send a letter to health care professionals mentioning the dangers, and work with Ortho McNeil, the company marketing the drug "tramadol," to develop new labeling that "discourages" prescribing it for high-risk patients.

At the same time, the FDA announced its investigation showed that "lindane," an insecticide used in prescription-only treatments for both lice and scabies, could cause neurological damage in children.

The danger was serious enough for the drug's label to warn parents that neurotoxicity (damage to nerves or nerve tissue) is possible among certain patients, especially infants.

Yet, the FDA will do no more than "recommended labeling changes that encourage lindane's use only for patients who have either failed to respond to adequate doses, or are intolerant of, other approved therapies."

In neither case did the FDA take any steps to withdraw the dangerous drugs from the market, or warn the public about the situation.

However, just one week later, that government agency began proceedings to ban sales of an herbal compound containing ephedrine. The targeted product, called "Herbal Ecstasy," is an herbal concoction which supposedly offers users a "natural high."

In a spectacular display of double standards, the FDA said it was not targeting the numerous prescription and over-the-counter (OTC) drugs containing ephedrine which are made by major pharmaceutical companies. Those drugs are often touted as weight loss aids, or treatments for asthma and allergies.

The then-FDA Commissioner David Kessler said of the Ecstacy compound, "I believe they're drugs and should be treated as such."

He gave no explanation as to why the herb was dangerous in the herbal supplement and not dangerous in the numerous OTC drugs sold to the public.

A spokesman for the manufacturer of Herbal Ecstasy denied that the product was dangerous, stating, "It's pretty silly that the FDA is trying to ban botanicals."

SOURCES: FDA Statement on Street Drugs Containing Botanical Ephedrine, April 10, 1996.

"FDA Requires Labeling Change on Lindane-Containing Lice Treatments," FDA news release, April 3, 1996.

"New Labeling for RX Pain Reliever, Tramadol," FDA news release, April 3, 1996.

"FDA warns consumers against products with ephedrine." The Associated Press, April 11, 1996.

FDA accused of protecting drug industry

For decades, Earl L. Mindell, Ph.D., has been considered one of the most respected authorities on health and vitamins. As the author of the classic "Vitamin Bible," as well as several other books, Dr. Mindell has led the campaign for better, safer foods and dietary supplements.

At times, it's been an uphill battle to convince people that vitamins and proper eating habits are more important to health than all the prescription and over-the-counter drugs put together.

A lack of accurate educational material, as well as constant attacks by the Food and Drug Administration (FDA) has slowed the public's acceptance of many natural remedies and health products.

According to Mindell, for the past 30 years, the FDA "has been out to destroy the vitamin and nutritional supplement industry. Look at the facts: FDA agents, with guns drawn, have raided health food stores and the offices of alternative physicians. They have harassed vitamin manufacturers. And they have launched a massive misinformation campaign of lies and scare tactics to discredit vitamins and nutritional healing."

Although the FDA claims to take such extreme measures out of its concern for public welfare, Mindell points to another possible motive.

"It's no coincidence that the FDA is intensifying its crackdown when vitamins, herbs, health foods, and natural remedies are reducing pharmaceutical profits. The FDA has long been the bodyguard of the medical establishment —

and particularly of the drug industry."

In a 1996 report, Mindell revealed that "The FDA receives large fees from pharmaceutical companies to have their drugs approved for public use. And the drug companies are only too happy to pay, since such approval guarantees them a legal monopoly for their new medications."

Prescription drugs represent a $56 BILLION market — and overall, drug prices went up 152% during the 10-year period from 1980 to 1990. With economic incentives like that, the drug companies have stepped up their assault, even going so far as to propose that some vitamin supplements be available on a "prescription only" basis.

"The FDA and the drug companies are doing everything they can to prevent you from learning about these safer, gentler (yes, and much cheaper) ways to heal and help yourself," Mindell warned.

To fight the FDA's protection of drug company profits, keep alert to proposed bills which would jeopardize your right to purchase vitamin or mineral supplements. Be ready to sign petitions posted at health food stores or alternative healing centers. Make sure your elected officials know you want an end to the medical-pharmaceutical monopoly!

SOURCE: *The Inside Story,* Spring 1996. "The Shocking Secret Story of Why The Government Wants to Ban Your Vitamins," by Dr. Earl Mindell.

FDA's boast about 'racing' to market

Before resigning as commissioner of the Food and Drug Administration, David A. Kessler, M.D., J.D., boasted that the FDA is winning the race to get drugs to the market quicker than Germany and Japan.

Sounding proud of revised procedures which some critics say placed speed before safety, Kessler reported on 214 products introduced into the world market from January 1990 through 1994.

Kessler also noted that the FDA had been criticized in the past for a "drug lag" which resulted in long delays between a product's approval abroad and its approval in the U.S.

After comparing how fast drugs were being rushed to the marketplace in each of several countries, Kessler and his colleagues reported, "When the analysis focuses on global drugs — those therapies approved in more than one of the four countries ... The U.K. and U.S. are a close first and second, and both clearly outpace Japan and Germany.

"For example," they continued, "41 drugs have been approved in three of the four countries. Of these, the U.K. was first to approve 39%, the U.S. was first to approve 37%, Japan was first to approve 15%, and Germany was first to approve 10 percent. The numbers are comparable for the 53 drugs that have been approved in either three or four countries... in many cases, the U.S. system allows priority drugs to reach consumers before they become more widely available."

The authors pointed to a Government Accounting Office (GAO) report showing that approval times of drugs by the FDA had been steadily decreasing for a number of years. After reviewing all drugs submitted to the FDA between 1987 and 1992, the GAO concluded that approval times had been reduced from an average of 33 months for drugs submitted in 1987 to an average of 19 months for drugs submitted in 1992. Approval times for priority drugs fell from 23 months in 1987 to 16 months in 1992.

The report did not address widely voiced concerns that, in its rush to approve drugs for sale by pharmaceutical companies, the FDA may be endangering the public. Determination of long-term results of drugs, critics say, is not possible in just 16 months.

SOURCES: Media advisory, American Medical Association and *The Journal of the American Medical Association (JAMA),* Dec. 10, 1996.

Device approved without long-term study

Most people feel uncomfortable talking about it, but urinary incontinence has become a major health concern in this country. An estimated 10% of all people aged 65 and over experience involuntary loss of urine — reflecting a higher percentage among women than men.

Studies have indicated that anywhere from 54% to 95% of people who use natural treatments (such as exercises) show significant improvement. Between 12 and 16% of them are cured entirely — without any risks.

Yet, this very common situation has become a cash cow for the medical and pharmaceutical industries. In 1987 alone, more than $10 billion was spent in drugs and surgery to correct incontinence.

In 1996, the FDA approved yet another medical device for use in treating urinary incontinence in adult women — despite a research study showing 44% of women who use it will probably develop urinary tract infections within the first year of use and 78% can expect to have some urethral discomfort and irritation, a problem so severe that it caused many women to drop out of the study. Other reported problems were bleeding and movement of the device into the bladder!

The device, available by prescription only, requires patients to be trained in its use by a medical physician. The device is inserted into the urethra by the user with a reusable syringe, and a balloon at the tip is inflated in the bladder to block leakage of urine. To urinate, the user removes the insert by pulling on an attached string to deflate the balloon. After voiding, the insert must be discarded and replaced with a new one.

In addition, patients are warned that they shouldn't wear the device for more than six hours at a time or during sexual intercourse and that use during pregnancy has not been studied.

The product was given an "expedited review" and the FDA's approval even though no studies had been conducted to determine the long-term rate of urinary tract infections or the effect of long-term use of the device on urethral tissue.

SOURCES: "Clinical Practice Guideline on Urinary Incontinence in Adults," The Agency for Health Care Policy and Research.

"FDA approves new incontinence product for women," Press release, UroMed Corp. August 21, 1996.

FDA jumping the gun

For years, drug and medical device companies complained that they couldn't put their products on the market quickly enough because the FDA took too long to approve them. Apparently, the FDA is now bending over backwards to please these firms. In 1996, it approved an application for an implantable heart device in only six days!

And, because the manufacturer had cut the five-year study short in order to market the product more quickly, the FDA didn't even have the complete research report to work with.

Then, the FDA beat its own record and approved a new drug in just FOUR DAYS — even though the drug's known side effects include diarrhea (in some cases, prolonged or severe enough to require treatment) and leukopenia, a temporary drop in white blood cells that reduces the body's ability to fight infections.

Despite the fact that research upon which the FDA based its sanction was so limited the agency warned approval might be withdrawn if post-marketing studies did not verify clinical benefits, the drug was approved for immediate use.

SOURCE: FDA Consumer, September 1996.

Big drug firms get U.S. Senate protection

In a vote taken June 27, 1996, the U.S. Senate took another step to protect the profits of multi-billion dollar drug manufacturers. At the urging of major firms such as Glaxo Wellcome, Inc., the legislators passed a bill that would delay the availability of lower cost generic drugs.

The vote ensured that the big-name, big-dollar drugs can retain their monopoly on the market, without competition from generic alternatives.

Glaxo Wellcome Inc., was singled out in many reports as a primary beneficiary of the vote, since its ulcer drug, Zantac — the world's top-selling drug — has a virtual strangle-hold on the market. In 1996, more than $2 billion was spent on Zantac in the United States.

In essence, the bill sanctioned the brand-name drug monopoly unless a generic manufacturer can show, in court, that it made substantial investments in the product and would pay royalties to the brand-name manufacturer.

To slip the bill past the Senate without attracting wide-spread public attention, the provision was tacked on as an amendment to a defense spending bill.

According to Sen. David Pryor of Arkansas, who supported a proposal that would allow generic drugs to be marketed more quickly, the vote translates into a "$2.5 billion windfall for Glaxo." Some observers are questioning possible economic motives behind the Senate vote.

In 1995, an article in *Congressional Quarterly*, raised the issue of conflict of interest. Specifically, it examined the case of Thomas J. Bliley, chairman of the House Commerce Committee, whose investment portfolio bulged with stocks from drugs manufacturers, as well as other companies influenced by House votes.

According to the article: "A review of Bliley's actions from 1990 through his first five months as chairman indicates that he has intervened with federal and local regulators on behalf of companies in which he holds stock. Bliley voted for legislation that would have directly benefitted a company in his portfolio, and he has sponsored amendments helpful to his investments."

In 1992, several major drug companies benefitted greatly from passage of a bill which extended their drug patents for two years. One of the companies affected was American Home Products, parent company of the ill-fated Dalkon Shield. Bliley's holdings in that company were estimated at between $50,000 and $100,000 and (not surprisingly) he voted in favor of the bill.

Although Bliley did not vote on the Senate bill, it is likely that numerous Senators involved in health care bills have similar personal interests in the outcome of legislation.

"Certainly," the *CQ* article concluded, "Bliley is not alone in holding stock in companies over which his committees have jurisdiction."

The *CQ* article also provided information on a study done by a university professor who reviewed the financial disclosure of Congressional members from 1991-93. The review showed that "83 made stock trades at the same time legislation affecting the companies in question was moving through Congress."

Three of those legislators were members of three committees with jurisdiction over health care reform and the trades involved companies in the health care field.

SOURCES: "Conflict of Interest Questions Raised by Bliley's Holdings," by David S. Cloud. *Congressional Quarterly*, May 30, 1995.

"Senate gives victory to brand-name drugs over generics." Associated Press. June 27, 1996.

Glaxo Wellcome's $2.1 million influence over congress

Health care advocates were shocked by the decision of the Food and Drug Administration (FDA) to allow drug makers to advertise prescription drugs on television giving only minimal information about the risks involved.

Many wondered why the U.S. government agency — which is supposed to protect the public from unsafe drugs and food additives — bowed to pressure from the drug industry, letting companies hawk their wares as though they were nothing more than a loaf of bread.

The reason appears clear in light of the amount of money drug firms spend each year in lobbying efforts.

Among the biggest of these is the gigantic Glaxo Wellcome company — the world's largest drug maker — which spent more than $2.1 million in the first six months of 1996 on congressional lobbying efforts. In addition to its five full-time lobbyists, it contracted with 50 more special interest advocates — including several former members of congress.

According to one investigative report, "The pharmaceutical giant has blossomed into one of the most influential companies in Washington."

Glaxo Wellcome pays for that influence by having its employee political action committee (PAC) give federal candidates huge donations, which have increased 400% in just the last 10 years. In fact, the PAC is so large that it is ranked 15th nationally.

But making contributions is only one way the company wins friends in congress. Another is by loaning or "renting" its 10-seat corporate jet to politicians, or providing other perks and favors.

Not everyone thinks the company is merely interested in improving the American system of government. Sen. Ted Kennedy once said that Glaxo was an example of corporate "greed."

In the report, published in the *Raleigh (N.C.) News & Observer,* Nancy Watzman, project director for the Center for Responsive Politics, a nonprofit campaign finance watchdog organization, said of Glaxo: "They're definitely very powerful. And they're doing all the things that make you powerful in Washington."

The report also revealed that, in 1989, Sen. Jesse Helms of North Carolina, "flew to Australia at Glaxo's request as part of the company's efforts to change a U.S. law that limited legal imports of Australian opium, a crop it controlled. A year later, Helms persuaded Congress to pass a $10 million tax break on import duties the company paid for an ingredient in one of its major drugs."

Glaxo has been able to dictate health care policy to congress as well, and was instrumental in defeating the reforms proposed by the Clinton administration.

In one of its larger moves, it put its weight behind the fight to save a 19-month patent extension passed as part of the 1994 General Agreement on Tariffs and Trade.

The extension meant that Glaxo's high-priced ulcer medicine, Zantac, would have no competition for nearly two more years. During that time, Glaxo could earn approximately $1 billion on the drug.

Critics in congress proposed an amendment that would have disallowed the patent extension. But, Sen. Orrin Hatch, R-Utah, stepped in and came up with a "compromise" which allowed Glaxo to keep it.

Was he acting out of a concern for public health and welfare? Possibly. Although the news report gave another possible motive.

Glaxo Wellcome had donated more than $20,000 to Hatch and his PAC since 1990. "The company also gave $5 million to the University of Utah's Huntsman Cancer Institute, which had been founded by a major Republican donor and Hatch supporter," stated *Raleigh News & Observer* investigative reporter Chris O'Brien. "Glaxo also flew Hatch here to give a speech to employees."

Other supporters of the pro-Glaxo bill had equally strong motives.

Lauch Faircloth, (R-N.C.) is a Glaxo stockholder and has received $15,000 in contributions from the company's PAC since 1990. Sen. Carol Moseley-Braun, D-Ill., received $9,999 in contributions and was paid twice to speak at Glaxo headquarters. Both signed a letter of support for the Hatch bill which was circulated to other senators.

The report included an interesting and revealing comparison made by the Center for Responsive Politics.

The 53 senators who voted in favor of Glaxo received an average contribution of $5,470. Those who voted against Glaxo received an average of $1,447. Ciba-Geigy, which fought against the patent extension because it wants to introduce a generic version of Zantac, donated an average of $578 to the 45 who voted against it.

After the smoke had cleared, Sen. Kennedy observed: "Corporate profits, not research and development, will be the prime beneficiary."

SOURCE: "Pharmaceutical giant swings heavy political stick," Chris O'Brien, *Raleigh News & Observer,* July 15, 1997.

Chapter 10

The "business" of sickness

I t is said that in early China, people paid their doctors on a regular basis —
as long as they remained heathy. If they got sick, the payments stopped
until the doctor helped them restore their health. After all, if they were ill
their doctor wasn't doing a very good job.

In modern America, our doctors get paid only if we get sick. If we were all
healthy, they would all be broke. To make money in medicine, one has to rely
on people getting ill — and staying that way.

This is not to suggest that medical doctors deliberately make their patients
sick. But there clearly is no incentive in our disease-treatment system to make
them healthy. In light of this reality, medical schools do not teach students how
to create health. They teach only how to suppress symptoms and treat disease.
At the very least, these are merely temporary "bandaids" which do nothing to
nurture lasting health.

Most hospitals and medical clinics are likewise geared to the profit-making
business of disease treatment rather than wellness. The end result is a health
care system which chooses expensive therapies over simple, inexpensive nutritional advice, and life-time medication routines over lifestyle changes.

Sickness a $425 billion business

According to a study in the *Journal of the American Medical Association*
(JAMA), a lot of people in America are sick — and they're making other
people rich.

An estimated 100 million Americans suffer from chronic health problems
such as cancer, heart disease, and arthritis — and they spend $425 billion a year
on drugs and surgery!

This may very well be at least part of the reason why the so-called "wars"
on cancer and other health problems have been such failures.

Despite massive fundraising efforts which pump billions of dollars into
medical research, experts agree that we are no closer to discovering a cure or
effective treatment in most cases. In fact, the *JAMA* study estimates that the
number of Americans with chronic conditions will increase to 148 million by
2030 and the direct costs — in 1990 dollars — will rise to about $798 billion.

One survey referred to in the study found that about 90 million Americans,
about 45% of the non-institutionalized population, suffered from one or more

chronic conditions.

The researchers said health care providers and policy-makers "must deal with how to transform our health care delivery system so that it better meets the needs of those living with chronic conditions."

They gave no suggestions, however, as to how the system might be transformed, particularly given the fact that there is a greater financial incentive to treat sick people than there is to keep people well.

SOURCE: "Persons With Chronic Conditions, Their Prevalence and Costs" by Catherine Hoffman, Sc.D.; Dorothy Rice; Hai-Yen Sung, Ph.D., *Journal of the American Medical Association,* Nov. 13, 1996.

Managed care systems accused of being heartless

Big medicine has become big business. That's the warning people got from the Consumer Attorneys Association of Los Angeles (CAALA), a health consumer advocacy group.

In a press release distributed in 1996, CAALA representative Chuck Mazursky explained that, "Managed care is the only business where you make money by turning away customers!"

Mazursky added that when HMOs deny care, injured patients and their families will be forced to take legal action. "Managed care is one more corporate enterprise, putting profits over patients. You can try to pass corrective legislation, but all too often there's only one thing that keeps big corporations honest: the threat of being taken to court."

First lady Hillary Rodham Clinton has already expressed concern that "managed-care companies are compromising the ability ... of physicians to exercise their professional judgment," Mazursky noted. "Even Speaker of the House Newt Gingrich said 'Any concentration of power in America has to be looked at. Clearly, health-maintenance organizations run by large insurance companies are concentrations of power'."

Managed-care questions are especially important in California, for several reasons:

➤ There are 13 million HMO members in California — more than in any other state;

➤ In Los Angeles, 61% of employees are in HMOs, compared with 27% nationwide;

➤ Six companies control 75% of the Los Angeles health care market; and

➤ Everything that happens in America happens in California first. "So, if we're the future of health care, what does that managed care future look like?," asked Mazursky. If the present is any indication, it will be a future where malpractice cases against HMOs will become commonplace.

To back up that prediction, he cited just a few of the instances of negligence and inhumane actions by HMOs:

❖ A stroke victim is denied needed medication by Health Net ... and suffers another, more severe, stroke that leaves her partially immobilized.

❖ A woman with a strange mole on her leg is twice denied a biopsy by her HMO ... for a growth that was a malignant melanoma.

❖ A man who sees blood in his urine is refused immediate treatment or referral by his HMO. After a two-week delay, the HMO performs the wrong test, without review or follow-up, and nine months later the man is diagnosed with bladder cancer.

❖ A wheelchair-bound attorney is forced into (the HMO) Kaiser Permanente by his employer. The HMO does not pay for the physical therapy he received under his private health care plan. The man, a paraplegic, develops an ulcerous sore on his buttocks but is never sent to see a specialist. When the sore ruptures and causes severe internal damage, the man is rushed to a private emergency room for a life-saving operation that the HMO refuses to pay for, calling it "not medically necessary." Kaiser paid only when threatened with a lawsuit.

"Patients need advocates in the HMO system," stated Deborah David of CAALA, "just like consumers do when corporations are deliberately negligent and make dangerous products, or when insurance companies deny legitimate claims. "This is different from medical malpractice," she added, "because the real problem in HMOs isn't the individual doctor. It's impersonal bureaucratic gobbledygook like 'capitation contracts' and 'utilization review committees' where corporate bean counters refuse to pay for treatment and constantly second-guess qualified doctors."

Even those doctors who want to act as advocates for their patients, are often prohibited from doing so, the CAALA release noted. According to an editorial in the *Los Angeles Times* (April 21, 1996) HMO doctors who speak out against the managed care system may violate "gag rules" and can be threatened with punishment, or termination. "In their harshest form, gag clauses explicitly prohibit doctors from telling patients the full range of treatment options," the *Times* stated.

It's become clear that big medicine is big business. Not long ago, Aetna bought U.S. Healthcare for $8.9 billion, and consumers could no longer ignore the fact that the practice of medicine is being taken over by big businesses with bottom-line corporate mentalities. As more and more people are forced into health-maintenance organizations, more and HMOs are denying them care ... in order to put money into their own pockets. Big business promises to cut costs. But does cost-cutting cost lives?

"We would prefer to have a health care system where saving money doesn't interfere with saving lives, where patients come first and legal action is never needed. But if it's up to consumer attorneys to keep the managed-care system honest and to ensure freedom of speech for doctors, we're ready," Mazursky concluded.

SOURCE:"Big Medicine, Bad Medicine," April 24, 1996, Consumer Attorneys Association of Los Angeles.

When profits come first, patients come last

Few people today would advocate a completely socialist health care system in the U.S., one in which all health care is paid for with tax revenues and doctors and hospitals are all non-profit enterprises.

However, the increased emphasis on the profitability of medical therapies — to the exclusion of concerns about their effectiveness — has a lot of people worried. Even some medical doctors are beginning to see that the profit motive driving the pharmaceutical and hospital industries can have a harmful effect on patient well-being.

Business and medical experts John H. McArthur, D.B.A. of the Harvard Business School and Francis D. Moore, M.D., Brigham and Women's Hospital, Harvard Medical School are authors of a detailed report on the problems faced in today's health care arena.

They stated that the purpose of their article — which appeared in *The Journal of the American Medical Association* — was to "explore threats to the quality and scope of medical care that arise when the tradition of medical professionalism is overtaken by the commercialism ethic and by corporations seeking profit for investors from the clinical care of the sick."

The authors cited a laundry list of potential hazards of the commercialization of medicine, including:

1. Diversion of funds. When a portion of funds for the care of the sick are diverted for corporate objectives (such as dividends, advertising, executive salaries), the resources available for health care are thereby reduced.

2. Risk avoidance. Exclusion of individuals and families from coverage because of prior disease, genetic constitution, predisposition, or high cost denies care to those most in need and is not a characteristic of national health insurance plans in other industrialized countries.

3. Downgrading of personnel. Highly qualified but expensive personnel will be threatened by discharge in favor of others with less experience and fewer credentials but lower income expectations.

4. Monopoly and loss of free choice. Free enterprise commerce fosters competition and encourages consumer choice among alternatives, but these choices cannot operate in rural areas, smaller communities, or inner-city areas where the population and financial resources are insufficient to attract more than a single prepaid health plan or HMO. Freedom of choice, long considered an ideal by-product of free competition, is compromised.

McArthur and Moore suggested that, "...minimum standards will be required to abate some of the hazards to society and abuses of patient care arising from commercial pressures on professional behavior."

In an accompanying editorial, Linda Emanuel, M.D., Ph.D., from the Ethics Institute, AMA, Chicago, wrote: "... unless investors in medical business can be held accountable for promoting medical professional standards, managers will always have an imbalanced motive to give priority to investment returns."

She added, "Professionalism requires restraints on profit-seeking activities, both as a moral matter and as a pragmatic one. The marriage of medicine with business is not optional. It is, for better or for worse, necessary. It is only a question of how constructively or destructively the two coexist, and some moderation in profit motive is a precondition for a constructive long-term partnership with medicine."

SOURCE: The Journal of the American Medical Association, (JAMA). March 25, 1997.

Insurance — not patient needs — often dictates cataract operations

When a patient undergoes an operation in a "fee-for-service" (FFS) setting, where the bill is paid either by the patient or the insurance company, the doctor usually gets far more money than when the patient is with a health maintenance organization (HMO).

It's not surprising, then, to find out that patients in FFS settings are **twice** as likely to be subjected to cataract operations than their HMO counterparts, according to an article in *The Journal of the American Medical Association (JAMA).*

Caroline Lubick Goldzweig, M.D., MSPH, from the Division of General Internal Medicine, Veterans Affairs Medical Center, West Los Angeles, Calif., and colleagues compared rates of cataract operations in two prepaid health settings and in traditional FFS settings.

The authors noted that patients in the traditional FFS system "had much higher rates of surgery than did those enrolled in staff-model HMO or independent practice association (IPA) settings."

The study included 43,387 staff-model HMO enrollees, 19,050 IPA enrollees, and 47,150 FFS beneficiaries. All the patients were Medicare beneficiaries aged 65 years and older.

The authors said the cataract extraction is one of the most common surgical procedures performed in the Medicare population, and accounts for Medicare's single largest expenditure.

The researchers explained that the difference in rates of cataract extraction could have a substantial impact on vision care for older persons. They added that their study did not try to determine the **need** for surgery across settings, but merely compared the frequency of the procedure under different paying situations.

The bottom line conclusion is that the decision to recommend surgery is often made not on what is best for the patient but on how much will be paid for the procedure.

The researchers noted that if cataract surgery is being underused in HMO settings because it's not as lucrative, "this would have important implications for visual disability, which if uncorrected, can lead to poor quality of life, greater risks for falls, hip fractures, and accidents, and may make cognitive function worse."

On the other hand, it's possible that too many people are being unnecessarily subjected to cataract surgery in FFS settings merely because it is a profitable and relatively risk-free procedure.

In an editorial appearing in the same issue of *JAMA,* Stephen A. Obstbaum, M.D., from the Department of Ophthalmology, Lenox Hill Hospital, New York, N.Y., added: "The variations in the frequencies of cataract extraction in the prepaid and fee-for- service settings should not be simply accepted as interesting statistics. Research that scrutinizes the reasons for these variations is warranted. Any system, whether prepaid or fee for service, should comply with the published standards that reflect what is in the best interest of the patient."

SOURCES: "Variations in cataract extraction rates in Medicare prepaid and fee-for-service settings," *The Journal of the American Medical Association (JAMA),* June 11, 1997.

"Should rates of cataract surgery vary by insurance status?" — editorial, *JAMA* June 11, 1997.

AMA loses credibility after selling name for endorsements

The Arthritis Foundation did it for a million dollars. Then the American Cancer Society got $4 million for doing it. No wonder the leaders of the American Medical Association (AMA) thought the group could pick up some easy cash by selling its name for "endorsements."

What they didn't count on was the tremendous public outcry which met the announcement that, in exchange for an undisclosed portion of the profits, the AMA would "endorse" a variety of home health products made by Sunbeam Corp.

The AMA and Sunbeam tried to convince the public that the arrangement was part of a public education program. In a press release distributed by Sunbeam in the summer of 1997, no mention was made of the compensation to be paid to the AMA for use of its name and logo.

Sunbeam's home health business includes nine product lines: heating pads, blood pressure monitors, thermometers, air cleaners, vaporizers, humidifiers, scales, hot & cold therapy and massagers. There was no indication that the AMA did any comparison testing to determine the value of these products or their superiority to others on the market. The decision to endorse them was based solely on the amount of money Sunbeam was willing to pay.

Al Dunlap, chairman and CEO of Sunbeam hinted at the true motives for the arrangement when he stated, "I expect that this alliance will further enhance our strong competitive position in the marketplace through expanding current distribution and gaining new distribution. ... This co-operative alliance will provide Sunbeam with a dramatic point of differentiation, versus our competition, as we will export the in-store merchandising concept internationally providing further strength to our brand leadership position."

But the public — and a large segment of the medical profession — was outraged that the AMA was willing to act as a marketing tool for a private company. What little credibility the AMA had left after years of missteps in the health arena suffered even more, as other medical organizations sought to distance themselves from the group.

The Massachusetts Medical Society (MMS) quickly issued a statement noting, "The Massachusetts Medical Society is no party of this agreement and had no prior knowledge of it. MMS is not an affiliate or local branch of the American Medical Association, although we are members of the same federation. The Massachusetts Medical Society is an independent medical organization and does not lend its official seal or name to the endorsement of commercial products, for financial gain or otherwise."

An editorial in the MMS publication, *New England Journal of Medicine (NEJM)*, criticized the AMA decision, stating, "Many physicians were embarrassed by the announcement of this ill-timed and ill-considered alliance, and we doubt whether the rank- and-file members of the AMA, if given the choice, would approve it.

"What's wrong with the arrangement? Plenty. It is one thing to recommend health-related products on the basis of careful scientific scrutiny; it is another to enter into an exclusive marketing arrangement with a single company in which royalties are linked to sales. An exclusive moneymaking deal of this kind seriously undermines the credibility of the AMA at a time when the public's trust in the profession has already slipped to dangerously low levels."

The authors, Jerome P. Kassirer, M.D., editor-in- chief of the *NEJM* and Marcia Angell, M.D., its executive editor, also questioned the AMA's right to pass judgement on Sunbeam items. They asked, "On what basis does the AMA claim to have expertise in assessing consumer products such as scales, air cleaners, massagers, and thermometers?"

In a surprising display of candor, Drs. Kassirer and Angell didn't stop at condemning the AMA, but blasted the entire medical profession for its growing greed and lack of ethics.

"Financial incentives are dangerous," they warned. "We have learned painfully that physicians respond to them. In a fee-for-service system they may order too many tests and procedures; in a capitated system they may order too few. When physicians have a stake in a laboratory, they send their patients there for studies, and when they have a financial interest in a hospital, they admit their patients there."

Their heavy guns, however, remained fixed squarely on the AMA.

"Membership is declining, and several of the organization's pronouncements about its goal of protecting patients and the physician-patient relationship over the past decade have been interpreted as disingenuous attempts to preserve the income of its members," they stated.

"Most recently, its support of the Partial-Birth Abortion Ban Act was widely interpreted as part of a deal with the Republicans in Congress to preserve Medicare billings for physicians. One had hoped for a new chapter in the

AMA's commitment to the public when it appointed a vice president for ethics standards only last year. Now," observed Kassirer and Angell, "it seems we are back to business as usual."

Acknowledging that other organizations are wallowing in the same mud as the AMA, they bluntly asked, "Why should the American Heart Association endorse only Bayer aspirin? And why should the American Cancer Society endorse only SmithKline Beecham's antismoking products? These organizations would do well to review the financial benefits of these associations against the potential blemishes to their reputations as keepers of the highest principles."

The MMS wasn't alone in its condemnation of the marketing agreement, and within days, the AMA issued a statement by Thomas R. Reardon, M.D., chairman of the AMA's Board of Trustees and P. John Seward, M.D., executive vice president, which admitted, "Our decision to approve the Sunbeam agreement in the form adopted was an error. As a result, our credibility was called into question."

In an attempt to repair the damage to its reputation, the AMA tried to change the conditions of the agreement. It still wanted Sunbeam to supply public educational material with its products, but said it would not "endorse" the products or accept money for the use of its name or logo.

Sunbeam wasn't pleased by the AMA's turnabout. It asked the Federal District Court in Chicago to enforce the terms of the five-year agreement. "The AMA cannot just change its mind and expect to walk away from our agreement because of adverse publicity directed at the AMA," Sunbeam Chairman Al Dunlap stated.

Regardless of court directives, it appears irreparable damage has been done. The AMA has shown itself to be interested more in its own financial welfare than in the public's health. In the future, its pronouncements about other medical issues — particularly concerning drugs and surgical procedures — will be even more suspect than they were in the past.

*SOURCES:*Statement: AMA Endorsement of Sunbeam Products, The Massachusetts Medical Society, August 15, 1997.

"The High Price of Product Endorsement," by Jerome P. Kassirer, M.D., editor-in-chief and Marcia Angell, M.D., executive editor, *The New England Journal of Medicine (NEJM)*, September 4, 1997.

"Sunbeam Corporation and American Medical Association Sign Exclusive Agreement," Press release, Sunbeam Corp., Aug 12, 1997.

"Sunbeam Asks Federal Court to Enforce AMA Contract," Business Wire, Sept. 8, 1997.

Statement by the American Medical Association, August 21, 1997.

Cancer Society image damaged by 'endorsement-for-pay'

Two consumer products received tacit endorsements from the American

Cancer Society (ACS), recommendations which could boost sales significantly. But many critics responded by saying the endorsements for NicoDerm anti-smoking patches and Florida orange juice were "bought and paid for."

According to an Associated Press (AP) article, the ACS was scheduled to receive an estimated $4 million for the use of its logo on product packaging and promotional material.

Paul Root Wolpe of the Center for Bioethics at the University of Pennsylvania condemned the arrangement.

"If they want to endorse products," he said, "they should do it in the spirit of an educational agency, not as a paid shill." Wolpe reasoned that non-profit organizations cannot provide objective information on health subjects if they are in business with companies that market products in those areas.

Quick to deny that it was selling approval of the products, the ACS stated: "The American Cancer Society does not formally endorse products. Our corporate partners are aware of this. We have formed educational and awareness-building partnerships with companies whose products match our established mission and which offer us the opportunity to reach people with ACS messages through media previously unavailable to us."

Disclaimer aside, critics worry that the Society's action marked the beginning of a growing trend of so-called "partnerships" between non-profit groups and companies. Since donations to many non-profit organizations are down — partly because people no longer believe there is a "medical" solution to all health problems — they are having to come up with other ways to raise funds.

This isn't the first time a major health organization came under fire for selling its name.

In 1994, the Arthritis Foundation was paid a million dollars by the makers of Tylenol for the right to use its name on product packaging. The agreement was clearly perceived by many consumers as an endorsement — a testimonial by the Foundation that Tylenol was somehow better than its competitors in combatting arthritis pain. In truth, the "endorsement" was based only on the exchange of money — not on any evaluation of the relative benefits of Tylenol.

The ACS claimed that it was "pursuing (these deals) because our constituents think it is the appropriate thing for us to be doing" — despite the fact that many people have been highly critical of the action.

SOURCES: Associated Press, "Cancer society endorsements spur debate," August 17, 1996.

"American Cancer Society Cause Related Marketing," American Cancer Society, August 20, 1996.

Drug company prosecuted for kickbacks, fraud

When patients go to medical doctors, they know they'll probably walk out of the office with a prescription in hand or a recommendation for additional health care services.

What they don't know is how the doctor made the decision about which medicine to prescribe or service to recommend. Most people assume physician decisions are based on experience, knowledge and the best interest of the patient.

Unfortunately, that's not always the case. Too often, M.D.s make their decisions based on a brochure left by a drug company's sales rep. Or even, in some cases, on kickbacks received from the company.

In one case prosecuted by the federal government, Caremark International, an Illinois-based drug manufacturer, was accused of paying kickbacks to physicians to get them to recommend their services, which included growth hormones and the administration of intravenous drugs to homebound patients.

Although the company refused to admit any wrongdoing, it agreed to pay $161 million in civil and criminal fines — as well as an additional $42.3 million to resolve "good faith business disputes" — and did plead guilty to two counts of mail fraud.

SOURCE: "Caremark to pay $42.3 million to settle all remaining fraud charges," Associated Press release, *American Medical News,* April 8, 1996.

Chapter 11

The "other" drug problem in America

W hat's the biggest health risk facing the average person today? No, it isn't cancer or heart disease. It's the side effects from medication. Prescription drugs can cause more health problems — and even death — than all the major diseases we worry so much about.

More than 90% of all office visits end in the doctor handing the patient at least one prescription (even if that visit was only lasted a few minutes) and seldom is the patient told about the dangers and side effects they present. Yet, every drug has side effects and most have a frighteningly long list of them. If as much attention were paid to the dangers of drugs as to their supposed "benefits," we would treat them with the same concern as we do loaded guns.

Prescription drugs kill 125,000 per year

According to a report from the National Pharmaceutical Council, some 125,000 deaths each year in the United States can be attributed to the improper administration of prescription drugs. In addition, failure of patients to take the drugs properly accounts for 10% of all hospital admissions, 25% of hospital admissions among the elderly, and 23% of all nursing home admissions. The national cost of this widespread prescription misuse exceeds $77 billion a year.

Many members of the medical establishment — which calls these tragedies "drug misadventures" — are quick to place the blame on pharmacists in an attempt to absolve themselves. One research study pointed out that fully one-third of the surveyed pharmacists failed to catch a potentially fatal prescription error.

Yet, some medical experts admit modern medical care is so rushed that doctors often do not exercise the caution needed when writing prescriptions. Instead of blaming pharmacists, they're looking for ways to have them shoulder more of the responsibility.

"In an age when physician visits are often limited to 10 or 15 minutes, pharmacists could play a valuable role in reinforcing instructions," noted an article in *American Medical News.*

SOURCES:"Pharmaceutical care touted as way to cut drug errors," by Sandra Lee Breisch, *American Medical News,* April 8, 1996.

"Drug-related morbidity and mortality: a cost-of-illness model," by Jeffrey A. Johnson and J. Lyle Bootman, Ph.D., *Archives of Internal Medicine,* Oct 9, 1995 v155 n18 p1949(8).

Prescription overuse a global problem

A report issued by the British Department of Health clearly shows that the problem of medicine overkill is not strictly an American phenomenon.

In 1995, according to the report, 473 million prescriptions were dispensed in England, reflecting an increase of nearly four percent over the previous year — averaging **nearly 10 items per person!** During the same period, the basic cost of prescription items dispensed was $3,681 million, marking an increase of just over eight percent.

SOURCE: "Department of Health Statistical Bulletin: Prescriptions dispensed in the Family Health Services Authorities; England 1985-1995," Department of Health, England.

Medication often masks warning signs

Keeping terminally ill patients comfortable makes sense, but medicating life's more common aches and pains often does more harm than good, stated an expert in pain management.

Pain clinics fill a specific role in caring for those suffering from cancer and other terminal diseases where comfort is a major goal of treatment. "But that is not where pain relief is for most of us," said James F. Fries, M.D., professor of medicine at Stanford University in Palo Alto, Calif.

"You do not want to risk your life treating minor symptoms," Dr. Fries observed in comments at the AMA's 15th Annual Science Reporters Conference.

Pain medication is taken for minor musculoskeletal problems more frequently than for anything else, Fries said in an interview. One example is non-steroidal anti-inflammatory drugs, or NSAIDs, taken by millions of Americans each day to relieve arthritis or muscular pain. Abdominal pain is a common side effect of NSAIDs, which cause one-third of bleeding ulcers.

"By taking a short term view of pain, one actually increases lifetime pain," according to Fries.

In addition, many NSAID users also take antacids to suppress the side effects of the drug, but wind up masking the very symptoms that would point to a bleeding ulcer.

"An excessive concern with pain relief gave us an epidemic of 10,000 to 20,000 deaths from bleeding ulcers each year, and hospitalizations from the same condition for another 100,000 to 200,000," Fries pointed out.

He argued that pain is an important defense mechanism that tells people to remove their hand from a hot stove or not to move an injured body part. In fact, he cited studies suggesting that low back pain responds best when you do nothing. Pain relievers allow muscles to relax, preventing back spasms that hold the spine immobile and prevent re-injury.

Fries deplored the attitude of people who make an appointment to see their physician and are often disappointed when told to skip the "heavy duty pain relievers" in favor of simply taking an aspirin. "We would like educated patients comfortable with their physician when he says to take acetaminophen, rather than the strong, dangerous stuff."

Exercise should play an important role in the coming environment of pain management, according to Fries. Once viewed as a form of beating up the body, research now shows that exercise and lack of pain go together.

"The role of exercise, the role of lifestyle, the role of psychological view toward pain and the role of an individual's pain threshold is the new integrated message," Fries said.

"Raising our pain threshold as an individual is one of the best things we can do for ourselves to reduce the need for pain medication." He mentioned marathon runners as one example of a group of people who have, through exercise, managed to raise their pain threshold.

Fries added that in pain management, "We have to change the emphasis of the problem, rather than focusing on tomorrow's pain level."

SOURCES:*Science News* press release, American Medical Association, October 2, 1996.

"Toward an epidemiology of gastropathy associated with nonsteroidal anti-inflammatory drug use," by James F. Fries. Medline record 89078928.

Many people still unaware of harmful effects of some pain medications

For years, non-medical health care providers have been warning patients about the potentially deadly side effects of many medications, especially pain pills. *Health Watch* provides scientific evidence about those risks in each issue.

Yet, many people still don't seem to realize that the medicine they are taking can cause far more problems than they're trying to "treat."

Even some medical doctors are echoing what health advocates have been saying all along.

A leading gastroenterologist joined the chorus by noting — somewhat belatedly — that people need to become aware that continually taking widely prescribed and over-the-counter medications for pain can lead to ulcers and other medical problems.

"It's a public health problem," stated Michael B. Kimmey, M.D., director of Gastrointestinal Endoscopy, University of Washington (Seattle) Medical Center, professor of medicine and assistant chief for clinical affairs, Division of Gastroenterology, University of Washington. Dr. Kimmey made the comments during an AMA media briefing on the complications of nonsteroidal anti-inflammatory drugs (NSAIDs).

Aspirin or other NSAIDs can be an ingredient in many over-the-counter (OTC) drugs, so some people may not even realize they're taking them. Dr. Kimmey said he would like to see pharmaceutical companies and the government both make an effort to help consumers become aware that they need to be cautious about these drugs.

"I think we need to have some responsible advertising. And we probably need to have that enforced by the Food and Drug Administration (FDA)," Kimmey stated.

Data from the Arthritis, Rheumatism and Aging Medical Information System indicate that approximately 76,000 hospitalizations occur each year from NSAID-induced gastrointestinal (GI) complications. Each hospitalization costs an average of $10,000.

Aspirin is the most familiar NSAID. NSAIDs also include ibuprofen, naproxen sodium and ketoprofen — each available in both prescription and OTC form — as well as a number of drugs available by prescription only. They are commonly used by millions of Americans to ease pain and in the case of aspirin, may also be prescribed for some cardiac patients.

A key problem, said Kimmey, is that many over-the-counter NSAIDs are taken by people who don't have a good reason to take them. "By doing so, people may," according to him, be "placing themselves at risk for a catastrophic problem."

In 1997, the FDA reviewed revised label applications from pharmaceutical companies which manufacture NSAIDs. The FDA sent letters to NSAID manufacturers after its Arthritis Advisory Committee unanimously recommended that all NSAID labeling be updated to include warnings regarding risk factors for severe GI complications.

Kimmey noted that people who take NSAIDs for several months may suffer any of three types of gastric side effects:

➤ *Dyspepsia* — Upper abdominal discomfort is common among people using these drugs. But most people who experience stomach aches do not develop ulcers.

➤ *Mucosal lesions* — These lesions are usually detected only through endoscopy, in which a lighted tube is passed into the stomach. Most people who develop these lesions do not have any symptoms.

➤ *Ulcers* — These are deeper sores or holes in the lining of the stomach or duodenum, and they may be accompanied by complications that include bleeding and perforation.

Kimmey pointed out that 50-80% of people who show up in hospitals suffering from gastrointestinal bleeding are taking NSAIDs. "Every time they come in with bleeding, they have a 10% chance of dying. I don't think people realize that until it may be too late."

SOURCE: Science News Update, July 16, 1997.

Top drug reference book filled with mistakes

It's considered the medical doctor's "drug bible" and is the primary source of information on the medicines which medical doctors prescribe for their patients. Yet, "The Physician's Desk Reference," better known as the "PDR," contains out-of-date and incomplete information on the management of drug overdoses.

That was the conclusion of researchers from the University of California

(USC), San Francisco School of Medicine who studied various entries in the book.

The "PDR," which is updated every year, is a compendium of the official FDA labelling for prescription drugs. Entries include information about each drug's chemistry, formulation, indications, dosages, and side-effects, as well as recommendations for the management of overdosage.

However, according to the USC researchers, the information it provides for handling overdoses is often wrong.

Entries for 20 drugs commonly involved in serious overdosages, including antidepressants, cardiovascular drugs, and analgesics, often recommended ineffective or contraindicated treatments or neglected to mention effective antidotes, the researchers pointed out.

"Of the 20 PDR entries, 16 (80%) had at least one deficiency, and five (25%) had two or more deficiencies ... three (15%) recommended contraindicated treatments."

In addition, the information is often contradictory, explained head researcher Walter Mullen. "If you look under procainamide, the PDR tells you not to use it for dig (digoxin) toxicity, but if you look under digoxin, it mentions using procainamide."

The publisher of the "PDR" tried to escape responsibility by saying that it only compiles the FDA-approved label information and makes no changes to it. Yet, the company failed to publicize, as was already noted in one research paper, that "The PDR is a collection of written and pictorial information that is provided and paid for by pharmaceutical manufacturers."

SOURCES: Archives of Internal Medicine, July 8, 1996.
Annals of Emergency Medicine 1997; 29: 255.61.
The Lancet, Feb. 8, 1997.

Cholesterol drugs pose risks

Researchers have released even more bad news about our fight against cholesterol: not only are the common tests unreliable, but the treatment — often unnecessary — carries significant risks.

According to a report by the British Department of Health, the number of people who are likely to be helped by cholesterol-lowering drugs is small — and numerous other reports say that the drugs may pose risk of increased cancer and other potentially deadly health problems.

In fact, the British researchers reported that only those individuals at "very high initial risk of coronary heart disease" had a chance of benefitting. Those at a lower risk level were actually more likely to die if they were treated with the drugs!

Luckily, most doctors no longer prescribe "clofibrate" — which used to be frequently given for cholesterol reduction — because it increased mortality rates from artery disease.

However, they continue to prescribe drugs like "cholestryamine," which has a long list of negative side effects, including a decrease in the ability of the blood to clot. Furthermore, animal studies have shown the drug to cause intestinal cancer. Also, this and other drugs have been linked to depressive illnesses, sexual dysfunction, skin rashes and digestive problems.

Many doctors are now questioning the need for such widespread cholesterol-lowering "therapy," noting that the level can be lowered too much, increasing the risk of cancer.

Unfortunately, since most medical schools do not provide adequate training in nutrition, M.D.s usually are unable to address the problem from that angle. They are taught to prescribe drugs or perform surgery and, as a result, that's the only thing many of them recommend.

As a result, prescriptions for cholesterol lowering drugs in some areas increased six-fold between 1986 and 1992.

SOURCES: *British Medical Journal,* May 22, 1993 v306 n6889 p1355(2). "The problem with cholesterol: no light at the end of this tunnel?" (Editorial by *Journal* staff).

British Medical Journal, May 22, 1993 v306 n6889 p1367(7). "Cholesterol lowering and mortality: the importance of considering initial level of risk."

The Lancet, March 21, 1992 v339 n8795 p727(3). "Low serum cholesterol and suicide."

Patient Care, March 15, 1996 v30 n5 p61(9). "Does reducing cholesterol improve CAD survival?" Includes related article on chances that lipid-lowering drugs may cause cancer.

Cancer Biotechnology Weekly, Jan. 15, 1996 p15(3).21 "Cancer risk warned from using cholesterol-lowering drugs."

American Medical News, Jan. 8, 1996 v39 n2 p56(1). "Cholesterol drugs tied to cancer in rats; link questioned."

The Journal of the American Medical Association, Jan. 3, 1996 v275 n1 p67(3). "Does lowering cholesterol cause cancer?"

Codeine doesn't work in many people

The pain-relieving drug codeine is totally ineffective in many people, according to findings presented at a national meeting of the American Chemical Society. The report showed a variety of differences in the drug's effectiveness and side effects, based on a person's ethnicity.

Researchers and physicians have long known that responses to any drug vary from person to person, and that some populations (the elderly, for example) can be more sensitive than others. Yet often, doctors have a "one size fits all" mentality when it comes to prescribing drugs.

Research presented at the 1997 meeting by Dr. Alastair Wood, a clinical pharmacologist at Vanderbilt University in Nashville, however, showed that codeine is unusual because the lion's share of its effect comes not from the drug itself, but from a substance the body makes from it.

That substance, or metabolite, is morphine, and the enzyme that manufactures it is called CYP2D6. Dr. Wood's research indicated that about 10% of Caucasians and 2% of Chinese lack this enzyme, and thus are unable to convert codeine to morphine to relieve their pain.

Although the drug has been prescribed to millions of patients for decades, this finding came as a surprise to researchers. That ignorance may have put many people at risk.

"Most drugs themselves produce the effect — so if a patient doesn't get the effect, the physician gives more of the drug," said Wood.

The research finding pointed out one of the many major dangers that exist with prescription drugs: the medical profession often has little or no understanding of the way they work or the long-term effect they may have on the body.

SOURCE:"Enzymes, Ethnicity Create Dramatic Differences in Codeine's Effectiveness in Humans," American Chemical Society, Sept. 5, 1997.

Prescription drug 'name game' has serious consequences

Each year, hundreds of new drugs are introduced — many of which have similar names. According to the Ontario Medical Association (OMA), "These look-alike and sound- alike drug names are a serious problem for physicians and pharmacists as they can cause confusion and potentially serious harm to patients."

As an example, the OMA pointed to a case in which a 79-year old man was given a prescription for Imferon (now discontinued in Canada), a drug used to treat iron deficiency. Yet, the pharmacist filled the prescription with the cancer drug *Intron*, which induced a fatal heart attack in the man. The pharmacist testified that the doctor's handwriting was difficult to read.

The problem is a major one in the United States as well.

In a Food & Drug Administration (FDA) bulletin report of medication errors which have caused deaths and injuries, that agency listed 15 pairs of drugs which were prescribed in error because of a mixup in similar-sounding drug names. For instance, drugs such as Norvasc and Navane, and Oruvail and Clinoril are causing a problem because of "similarity when handwritten," the FDA noted.

The FDA also reported that a drug called Flumadine, which is used in the treatment of illness caused by various strains of influenza-A, "has been inadvertently given to several patients instead of EULEXIN (Flutamine) which is used to treat prostate cancer."

In the same bulletin, the FDA called doctors' attention to several "fatalities which were reported from inadvertent administration of excessive doses of concentrated Epinephrine Injection." The FDA pointed out that "because of the wide range of epinephrine-containing injectable products on the market, confusion is possible, especially in an emergency."

Although stating point-blank that "medication errors can be a source of significant morbidity and mortality in the health care setting," the FDA failed to alert both the drug-dispensers and the drug takers with a strongly worded warning. Instead, the report ended with a standard cautionary note: "We encourage confirmation of the patient's diagnosis before dispensing the above medications as one means of reducing the potential for a medication misadventure."

The term "medical misadventure," is a phrase often used by the medical community to refer to a drug error which can seriously injure or kill a patient.

SOURCES: FDA Medical Bulletin, June 1996, Vol. 26, No. 2.

"The Coroner's Inquest," Ontario Medical Association Drug Report, June 1995.

Diet and nutrition key factors in health — but few medical schools teach it

Most Americans regard their medical physician as their primary source for reliable nutrition advice. Yet, most M.D.s have little or no training in nutrition. The Association of American Medical Colleges reported that in 1995, only 29 out of 129 U.S. medical schools (fewer than 23%) had a required nutrition course. Thirty-two schools (nearly 25%) offered no nutrition education at all.

"Nutrition is now recognized as a key modality for health promotion and disease prevention in the 21st century. Still, education of physicians on nutrition-related matters is abysmal," stated Richard Deckelbaum, M.D., director of the Institute of Human Nutrition at Columbia University.

One study found that only *six percent* of medical students took advantage of an elective nutrition course when it was offered. Frequently, medical students aren't even aware of the elective or its significance in a clinical setting.

"I graduated from medical school in 1963 and back then they didn't realize the importance nutrition played in many of the major diseases such as cancer and diabetes. It didn't seem as important then to include courses on nutrition," said Dr. Mohammed Khonsary, a private practice internist in New Jersey and student of the program.

"It would be wise now to place a greater emphasis on nutrition," he continued, "such as the broad role fruits and vegetables play in disease prevention, and include more classes on the subject, especially since we now have 60 million overweight people in this country."

Dietetics has a venerable history in medicine that stretches back at least to Hippocrates, who regarded it as virtually inseparable from medicine. In fact, four of the 10 leading causes of death in the United States are diet-related conditions: diabetes, heart disease, stroke and cancer.

So, when did physicians lose site of nutrition's role in health?

"Clinical nutrition has been overlooked because it cannot be identified with any particular physiological system in the body, as most medical specialities can," said Dr. Deckelbaum.

He added that better nutrition can result in delaying the onset of many chronic diseases, such as heart disease or cancer, by five years or more, a factor that will decrease health care costs in the United States by more than $80 billion annually.

Not all medical doctors seem to be aware of this — or care.

The Institute of Human Nutrition at Columbia University College of Physicians & Surgeons has developed a master of science degree in nutrition for practicing physicians. The program offers physicians an opportunity to augment their training with a foundation in basic and clinical nutritional sciences. Just **seven** doctors enrolled in the program when it was introduced.

SOURCE: "What Role Does Diet Play in Health and Disease Prevention? Surprise! Many Physicians May Not Know," College of Physicians and Surgeons at Columbia-Presbyterian Medical Center Office of Public Health, April 17, 1997.

Using asthma inhalers may lead to glaucoma

Prolonged use of high doses of inhaled steroids may increase the risk of glaucoma or ocular hypertension, cautioned Canadian researchers who studied more than 48,000 patients.

Edeltraut Garbe, M.D., from the Royal Victoria Hospital, McGill University Health Centre, Montreal, Canada, and colleagues studied the relationship between the use of inhaled and nasal steroids and glaucoma in 48,118 patients in the Quebec universal health insurance program for the elderly.

The authors said the increase in glaucoma was noticed in patients who took a high dose (1,500 micrograms or more of the inhaled steroid flunisolide, or 1,600 mcg or more of the other inhaled steroids) for three months or more.

The risk for glaucoma was 44% higher for those who used high doses of inhaled steroids for three months or longer compared with nonusers. It has been estimated that in excess of eight million prescriptions were written worldwide for nasal steroids in 1993, according to the researchers.

Ocular hypertension is high pressure within the eye that can result in partial or complete loss of vision.

In recent years, there has been a trend to prescribe higher doses of inhaled and nasal steroids. However, researchers have begun to raise concerns over possible adverse effects of these drugs, the report stated.

The authors stated: "The results of our study should alert physicians to the possibility that inhaled steroids may cause ocular hypertension and open-angle glaucoma, especially when they have been administered in high doses over extended periods of time. The use of these drugs should be routinely questioned in newly diagnosed cases of ocular hypertension and open-angle glaucoma," they said.

"If patients receive high doses of inhaled steroids over several months, ocular pressure should be monitored. Further research is needed to investigate the clinical course of ocular hypertension and open-angle glaucoma associated with inhaled glucocorticoids," they concluded.

SOURCE: The Journal of The American Medical Association (JAMA), March 4, 1997.

'Safe' treatment for migraine can cause addiction

Medical doctors rarely criticize drugs or drug companies in public, partly because they have been taught to revere "miracle" drugs and partly because a great deal of their income depends on their alliance with the firms.

But sometimes, tragedy strikes home, causing an M.D. to break ranks and unveil the less-than-miraculous side effects of some commonly prescribed medications.

Such was the case with neurologist Morris A. Fisher, M.D., professor of neurology at Loyola University, Stritch School of Medicine, Maywood, Ill. After his son committed suicide during treatment for an addiction to a supposedly "safe" treatment for migraine, Dr. Fisher and his niece, investigative reporter Stephanie Glass, Fairfield, Conn., gathered information on the drug through the Freedom of Information Act.

The results of Fisher's investigation were published in the research journal, *Neurology.*

According to Fisher, medical professionals and patients are not being informed or warned about the serious dangers associated with the nasal spray *Stadol* (generic name, "butorphanol") which is delivered as a nasal spray.

The lack of information on the increasing incidence of addiction/dependence associated with Stadol, manufactured by Bristol-Myers Squibb, is largely due to the failure of the Food and Drug Administration (FDA) to identify and act on the abuse potential of the drug and to recommend further controls to the Drug Enforcement Administration (DEA), according to the journal article.

Fisher stated that evidence showing abuse potential should force the FDA to recommend to the DEA that the drug be *scheduled.* Drugs which are scheduled are controlled by the DEA because of their potential for dependence. These drugs are much more closely tracked to prevent diversion into illegal channels.

Medical evidence, said Fisher, has always indicated that Stadol, a synthetically derived opioid, is an addictive drug that should be scheduled for both effective control and as a caution to physicians and patients.

"The failure to do this has caused considerable harm and repeated the well-established pattern of narcotic drug use in the United States," Fisher wrote, noting that this evidence has been accumulating for a long time.

In 1978, as part of the drug approval process, the FDA's Drug Abuse Advisory Committee (DAAC) reviewed an injectable form of Stadol. The committee recommended scheduling Stadol pointing out its abuse potential and withdrawal symptoms in people who had received the drug during clinical trials. The committee's recommendation was not followed.

Arguments against scheduling the drug included **patient convenience** and **decreased commercial potential.**

Soon after the approval, reports were made to the FDA of abuse and adverse drug reactions including psychological disturbances consistent with narcotic use — confusion, hallucinations and paranoid reactions.

During the period 1979-92 adverse drug reactions from Stadol were reported to the FDA at a rate of about 60 per year, six of which annually were reports of dependence/addiction, and one death. However, since the drug was largely administered within the confines of hospitals or clinics, "interpretation of these reports was that they were not of 'very great significance.'"

In 1989, Bristol-Myers Squibb, applied for approval of Stadol as a nasal spray. The DAAC again discussed the issue of scheduling the drug, including the likelihood of increased abuse potential due to the nasal spray form.

In the record of the approval process, Fisher found that the manufacturer argued there was no new evidence for potential or actual abuse. However, the record also contains evidence for physical dependence on Stadol with rats, monkeys, baboons, and humans. The FDA review panel's conclusion, according to Fisher, was to wait to see if problems arose.

Despite the fact that the drug maker told the FDA that Stadol would not be used chronically, Fisher reported that in 1991 after the nasal spray form of the drug was approved, the company's advertising campaign promoted its use for migraine headaches, "a condition in which repeated long-term use could be anticipated."

Stadol was promoted in advertising materials as a safe pain killer for migraines, with few and minor side effects. Fisher pointed out that the relatively mild side effects mentioned in Bristol-Myers Squibb product literature stood in stark contrast to the reality.

The documents he uncovered show that during the first three years after release of the nasal spray, adverse drug reactions reported to the FDA increased from "60 per year to about 400 per year." About half were major psychological disturbances or dependence/addiction.

Fisher said that physicians rely on the DEA to control addicting prescription drugs and the FDA to keep them informed. "The fundamental issue raised by the history of (Stadol) use is the lack of accurate and timely information," he stated.

"For example, that dependence/addiction is by far the most common adverse effect of a drug reported to the FDA is obviously important medical information, but the public is not well-served if meaningful drug information can be obtained only through the Freedom of Information Act."

Concluded Fisher, "The experience with Stadol should not be repeated."
SOURCE: Neurology, May 1997.

Medical doctors ignore warnings about dangers of Prozac

We've been called the "Prozac Nation," and the term isn't much of an exaggeration. About 43 million prescriptions for anti-depressants like Prozac were written in 1995 — with children as young as five-years-old being pumped full of the drug.

The situation is frightening and getting worse. Even the media — known more for its praise of the medical profession — has tried to alert the public.

The *U.S. News and World Report,* warned that, "Perhaps tens of thousands of kids are being given the medication (Prozac) — and the lesser-known Zoloft and Paxil — despite a lack of scientific proof that these drugs are safe and effective for children."

The problem hasn't only been occurring in the United States. The popular Canadian magazine *Maclean's,* reported, "Many medical experts worry that some doctors may be overprescribing Prozac and using it to treat relatively trivial personality disorders."

But doctors haven't been using Prozac only as a "happy" pill. They've been prescribing it for a multitude of symptoms.

"In 1987, for example, a year before Prozac was approved for alleviating depression, scientists observed that many patients lost weight while taking the drug. Word got out, and now some physicians prescribe Prozac to treat obesity as well," noted *Time* magazine.

Maclean's added: "In Canada and the United States, Prozac has been approved for use in treating clinical depression, bulimia (habitual purging to lose weight) and obsessive-compulsive disorder (persistent irrational thoughts and actions). But many doctors have effectively expanded the definition of what constitutes clinical depression to include dysthymia — chronic low-grade depression — and in some cases have prescribed Prozac to otherwise healthy patients suffering from low self-esteem or gnawing anxieties. Hubert Van Tol, an associate professor of psychiatry and pharmacology at the University of Toronto, says: 'If it's a question of someone who isn't feeling so hot, or maybe a man who's nervous about addressing meetings — that's not what the drug was designed for.'"

Even the strongest supporters of anti-depressants like Prozac would agree that doctors need to make a very careful diagnosis before prescribing the drug.

As was reported in *Redbook* magazine, "Patients must be carefully diagnosed to pinpoint their disorder as true depression rather than manic depression or another condition that Prozac might aggravate. 'If they have a family history or a propensity for it, Prozac is no different from any other antidepressant in its capacity to flip people into mania [the *up* stage of depression],' Dr. (Frederick) Goodwin says.

"'It can also produce anxiety, and if a person is already suicidal, getting suddenly anxious could push her over the edge.'" Dr. Goodwin is head of the Alcohol, Drug Abuse, and Mental Health Administration of the Public Health Service and the government's top psychiatrist.

Yet, a Rand Corporation study discovered that doctors prescribe such anti-depressants after an average of only three minutes of conversation!

While thousands of patients swear Prozac saved their lives, it is far from being a miracle drug. It has been implicated in numerous suicides and acts of violence, and can cause nausea, nervousness and insomnia. But those are the tip of the iceberg.

In the *Maclean's* article, Dr. Lorne Brandes, a Winnipeg cancer researcher, stated there was evidence that Prozac and some other widely used drugs may promote the growth of cancerous tumors.

"I'm very concerned about Prozac," said Brandes, whose 1992 research showed that rats and mice with artificially induced cancer showed an increased rate of tumor growth when they were given Prozac and another antidepressants.

Cancer may not be the only danger lurking the streets of the Prozac Nation.

Sidney Wolfe, director of the Public Citizen Health Research Group, a Washington-based consumer advocacy organization, compares Prozac to Valium. The popular tranquilizer was sold for more than a decade before doctors realized it was extremely addictive. "Prozac," declared Wolfe in the *Maclean's* report, "has become the Valium of the 1990s."

Why, then, hasn't the drug been yanked off the shelves? The answer is clearly written in the financial report of its manufacturer, Eli Lilly.

According to *Money* magazine, "Prozac had a cheery year in 1995, with sales for the antidepressant topping $2 billion. Those figures have perked up profits at Eli Lilly, the $7.2 billion pharmaceutical company located in Indianapolis. As Lilly's star product, Prozac has accounted for upwards of 40% of the company's recent growth." Projected sales for 1996 topped $2.4 billion.

But even though health care experts are worried that the drug may be killing us and our children, company officials are smiling.

"Since Prozac is so well established, the drug is *at the most profitable part of its life cycle,*" said stock analyst Steve Buell in the *Money* article. He points out that "with no new advertising, sales efforts or research needed, the margins on any additional sales could be as high as 99%."

Not everyone is smiling along with the company, which has been accused of underhanded tactics to suppress information about the true dangers of the drug.

"What is distressing is the fact that a significant number of people do have very bad reactions to Prozac, chiefly suicidal impulses ... and it is Lilly's concerted efforts to minimize such sinister side-effects that remain even now indefensible," said famed author William Styron, in *The Nation*.

"Meanwhile," he continued, "the advisory committee of the Food and Drug Administration that was organized to study Prozac — five of whose eight members, according to (Alexander) Cockburn had financial backing from Lilly — gave the medication its O.K."

The dirty dealings even reached the legal arena.

In December 1994, Eli Lilly triumphantly announced it had won a court case involving a man who killed eight people, injured 13, then committed suicide. He had started taking Prozac one month before his violent outbreak and both his family and his victims argued that the company had not properly warned people about the possible dangerous side effects of the drug.

However, a report in the *Jersey Law Journal* a short time later revealed several facts which were not disclosed by Eli Lilly.

The company had entered into a settlement with the plaintiffs **before the case went to the jury!** Part of the secret settlement called for the plaintiffs to keep quiet about previous, similar activities by Eli Lilly. In court, no one heard the evidence that the company, a decade earlier, had failed to report adverse reactions to another one of its drugs - - which was later linked to the deaths of more than 100 patients.

John Potter, the judge in the 1994 case, explained that, "On December 8, 1994, after a day's delay at the parties' mutual request and without explanation, the plaintiffs elected not to introduce the evidence they had fought so hard to get admitted. The jury ultimately returned a verdict for Lilly." After finding out about the secret agreement between the plaintiffs and the drug maker, Potter stated that his ruling should be changed from not guilty to "dismissed as settled."

SOURCES:"Smile with Prozac — and laugh to the bank with Eli Lilly," by Duff McDonald. *Money,* April 1996 v25 n4 p88(1).

"Anti-depressants have uses, but they're used by too many," by Steve Wilson. *The Arizona Republic,* June 5, 1996. pA2.

"Kindergartners in the Prozac nation: are there risks in giving kids antidepressants?" by Beth Brophy. *U.S. News & World Report,* Nov. 13, 1995 v119 n19 p96(2).

"Double-duty drugs: approved medications are being widely prescribed for unapproved uses," by Christine Gorman. *Time,* Sept. 18, 1995 v146 n12 p96(2)

"Questioning Prozac: are too many people popping a pill to treat clinical depression?" by Mark Nichols and Patricia Chisholm. *Maclean's,* May 23, 1994 v107 n21 p36(4).

"Prozac days, Halcion nights: profits and pills," by William Styron. *The Nation,* Jan. 4, 1993 v256 n1 p1(4).

"Beat the Devil" by Alexander Cockburn. *The Nation* December 7, 1992.

"The secret deal that won the Prozac case," by M. Castellano. *Jersey Law Journal,* May 1, 1995.

"Eli Lilly and the FDA," by Dr. Gary Null. *Townsend Letter for Doctors,* Mar. 1993, 115/1616:1, 178-187.

Pharmacists failed to notice fatal prescription error

After surveying 50 Washington, D.C. pharmacies, researchers at Georgetown University Medical Center found that nearly one-third of retail pharmacies failed to detect a potentially life-threatening prescription error.

The study, conducted by John Cavuto, M.D.; Raymond Woosley, M.D., Ph.D.; and Mark Sale, M.D., Departments of Medicine and Pharmacology, appeared in a letter to the editor in the April 10, 1996 issue of the *Journal of the*

American Medical Association.

The findings suggested that more effective safeguards were needed in medical and pharmacy communities to prevent human prescription errors, and that computerized drug-interaction screening programs intended to correct such errors may be less effective than previously thought in deterring prescriptions of potentially dangerous drug combinations.

Realizing that physicians can mistakenly prescribe drugs that have the potential to interact, the Georgetown researchers visited the Washington metropolitan area pharmacies to determine whether the pharmacist would simultaneously fill prescriptions of two interacting drugs — "erythromycin" and "terfenadine" (also known by its brand name Seldane).

Although the two medications are very commonly prescribed drugs, they can cause a potentially fatal heart arrhythmia if taken together.

The researchers considered pharmacies effective in deterring the prescription error if the pharmacist refused to fill the prescription — or agreed to fill the prescription, but advised the patient to not take the two medications together, or call his or her physician first.

Sixteen of the 50 pharmacies (32%) filled the two prescriptions without comment. Forty-eight of the 50 pharmacies had computer programs in use designed to prevent drug interactions from occurring. Fourteen of these 48 pharmacies (29%) failed to detect a prescription error.

"Our survey shows that better systems and greater educational efforts are needed for both physicians and pharmacists to prevent prescription errors," said Woosley, chairman of the Department of Pharmacology. "It seems clear that a computer system alone isn't enough without some informed human intervention. Ongoing educational programs are required to educate health care providers and the public about drugs."

Each year more than two billion prescriptions are written, amounting to an average of about eight prescriptions per person. In the elderly, the average is 15 per year, per person. Prescribing errors are the second greatest cause of medical malpractice in the United States today.

Woosley has championed the creation of a federally-funded Centers for Education and Research in Therapeutics that could address the information gap on medications.

"Science is not perfect and never complete," Woosley added. "It needs to be interpreted thoughtfully, and the art in medicine occurs when you, as a physician, as a pharmacist, or as a consumer, know when to ask questions, when to seek more information, when to be cautious, and when to seek a broader base of knowledge."

"As a society, we know very little about the numerous medications we are taking," continued Woosley. "There is room for improvement in therapeutics in the medical community and consumers should make it their prerogative to have educated, informed people involved in their healthcare to be guaranteed safety."

SOURCE"Greater safety measures needed in pharmacies to prevent prescription errors, study finds," Georgetown University Medical Center, April 9, 1996.

Antihistamine drugs linked to heart abnormalities, death

Just months after the Food and Drug Administration (FDA) approved a non-sedative antihistamine which claims to be safer than the controversial "terfenadine" (marketed under the trade name *Seldane*), a Swedish drug monitoring center warned that "the data indicate that some of the alternatives to terfenadine may have similar problems."

According to the FDA, terfenadine was introduced in 1985 and was supposedly the first prescription antihistamine to relieve the symptoms of hay fever without causing drowsiness. But the drug did more than just stop people's sniffles — it stopped their hearts.

The FDA received reports of serious — sometimes fatal — cardiac arrhythmias associated with terfenadine when it was taken with a number of other commonly prescribed medications or by patients with liver disease. These other drugs, such as "erythromycin" (an antibiotic) and "ketoconozole" (an antifungal drug), can cause terfenadine build up in the blood and result in serious cardiac side effects.

Despite the fact that the drug could kill, the FDA refused to take it off the market, asking only that the drug maker warn doctors and pharmacists of the dangers involved.

However, an investigative report shown on the January 14, 1997 episode of the Canadian Broadcast System's "Market Place," revealed that patients were often not warned of the risks. The show sent people undercover to 70 different drug stores in seven major cities. At more than half (36) of the stores, the "patients" were never asked about other drugs they were taking, or warned of the dangers.

"We were so taken aback by those results we decided to do a second survey in one city only, in Toronto. And this time we took a hidden camera along," the producers explained.

"We found the consumer well served by some pharmacies. But in the majority, the only question we were asked was what size we wanted. In our second survey, we went to 45 pharmacies. We were given no warnings at 28 stores."

More than 14,000 prescriptions for Seldane continued to be filled every year and the reports of cardiac irregularities continued. Yet, the FDA decided that "the agency considered the benefits of terfenadine to outweigh its risks despite its known serious cardiac adverse effects when used inappropriately." Translation: suppressing the symptoms of hay fever was worth risking a fatal heart abnormality caused by the drug.

In early 1997, however, the FDA said it was considering withdrawing its approval of Seldane, not because of any new evidence or a heightened concern for public safety, but because the drug company had managed to produce a substitute drug, called *Allegra,* to replace the profitable Seldane.

"Now that Allegra is available and provides the therapeutic benefits of terfenadine without the associated serious cardiac risks, terfenadine's benefits are no longer considered to outweigh its risks," the FDA announced.

But is the new drug really safer? That's the question being asked by researchers around the world.

The new report, issued by the Swedish drug monitoring center operated by the World Health Organization (WHO), did not specifically name Allegra, but concluded that, "the data indicate that some of the alternatives to terfenadine may have similar problems, suggesting that thorough consideration of the comparative benefit risk profile of all non-sedating antihistamines is wise."

SOURCES: The Lancet, May 3, 1997.

"FDA Proposes to Withdraw Seldane Approval," *FDA Talk Paper,* Jan. 13, 1997.

Press release, Georgetown University Medical Center: "FDA approves safer version of Seldane developed by Georgetown pharmacologist."

"Market Place," Canadian Broadcast System, January 14, 1997.

M.D.s still prescribing potentially deadly drug combination

Since 1990, medical doctors and pharmacists have been warned that taking the prescription antihistamine terfenadine ("Seldane") along with a certain type of antibiotic or antifungal medication could cause life-threatening side effects.

Still, many doctors continue to prescribe the two drugs at the same time, according to an article in *The Journal of the American Medical Association (JAMA).*

David Thompson, Ph.D., and Gerry Oster, Ph.D., Policy Analysis, Inc., Brookline, Mass., reviewed computerized pharmacy claims from a large health insurer in New England between January 1990 (six months before the first warning was issued) and June 1994.

They checked first for patients with paid claims for terfenadine, then cross-checked to see if any of them had also been given prescriptions for the antibiotics or anti-fungals at the same time.

The researchers noted that although there was a decline in the number of "same-day" prescriptions, "as many as 2-3 percent of all persons prescribed terfenadine had overlapping claims for either a macrolide antibiotic or imidazole antifungal." Both of those drugs could, when taken with terfenadine, cause severe side effects — even death.

The researchers wrote: "Some persons actually had more than one such claim associated with a given prescription for terfenadine. Concurrent use of terfenadine and contraindicated drugs therefore may remain a problem, and substantial numbers of persons may be at elevated risk of serious drug-drug interactions."

In June 1990, the U.S. Food and Drug Administration (FDA) issued a report warning that the drug combination could cause ventricular arrhythmias. In August 1990, the FDA ordered the manufacturer of terfenadine (Hoechst Marion Roussel) to send a "Dear Doctor" letter to all practicing physicians in the U.S. alerting them to this problem. In July 1992, warning labels were added to all products containing terfenadine.

In addition, the study says providers have been alerted to the possibility of drug-drug interactions involving terfenadine through publication of case reports, warnings, commentaries, and clinical investigations.

Concluded the researchers: "Despite substantial declines following reports of serious drug- drug interactions and changes in product labeling, concurrent use of terfenadine and contraindicated macrolide antibiotics and imidazole anti-fungals continues to occur."

SOURCES: "Use of terfenadine and contraindicated drugs," *The Journal of the American Medical Association (JAMA)*, May 1, 1996 v275 n17 p1339(3).

"Potentially deadly combination of drugs still prescribed and dispensed," AMA Media Advisory, April 30, 1996.

Many medications can have negative side effects on gums

People are gradually becoming aware that common prescription and over-the- counter drugs can have serious negative effects on their health.

According to Sebastian Ciancio, D.D.S., a clinical professor of pharmacology and professor of periodontology at the University at Buffalo School of Dental Medicine, those same drugs can cause dental problems as well. Dr. Ciancio presented findings of his research at the American Dental Association's (ADA) 138th Annual Session on Saturday, Oct. 18, 1997.

Of primary concern are the more than 400 medications that can cause "dry mouth," which, in turn, can cause a number of dental problems.

In addition, Ciancio listed three types of medications that have been shown to cause swelling in the gums:

➤ calcium channel blockers, used to treat high blood pressure or cardiac arrythmia;
➤ anti-convulsive medications such as dilantin, used to treat conditions such as epilepsy; and
➤ drugs (cyclosporin) used by patients who have received liver, kidney or heart transplants.

The problem with these medications is that as they cause the gums to swell. The gum disease has larger crevices to set up shop in and spread to underlying bone, causing severe periodontal disease and bone loss.

SOURCE:"Medications Have Unintended Positive and Negative Side Effects on Gums," American Dental Association, October 18, 1997.

Chapter 12

No 'safe' drugs

E ven people who realize that prescription drugs can be dangerous are often lured into thinking that over-the-counter (OTC) drugs are "safe." After all, would the FDA really allow dangerous or ineffective medications to be sold to the American public? Yes, they do! And they fail to regulate any but the most extreme abuses by drug companies.

A Senate investigation on over-the-counter drugs once concluded that the majority of these medications were completely useless, and most posed at least some health dangers. But it didn't change the pharmaceutical industry or even the regulations which are supposed to keep the drug companies in line.

Since neither they nor the government will do it, it's up to the American people to protect themselves from these unsafe medications by reading the facts and changing the way they think about health care. It won't be found in capsule form on any drug store shelf.

Aspirin makers continue to deceive public

Television commercials have tried to reinforce the image of aspirin as "preventive medicine," saying that taking aspirins regularly can protect against heart attack.

For their "proof," they've pointed to a 1988 medical study, featured in the *Journal of the American Medical Association (JAMA)*, containing the preliminary results from a controlled experiment of **high-risk** men. The study found that the men who took aspirin had half the number of heart attacks as those in the group that didn't take it.

But, the study also found that those taking the aspirin suffered more strokes!

Because of this, and because of admitted limitations in the study's methodology the *Journal* editor and the report's authors concluded that the public should *not start taking aspirin* to prevent heart disease.

Based largely on press releases distributed by aspirin makers, the media made a big story of the study, often totally misrepresenting it.

"The possible implications of the manner in which the five largest newspapers reported the study are such that individuals may have started taking aspirin regularly to prevent heart attacks, a practice which can lead to serious health consequences such as strokes," said researcher Fred Molitor, who holds a Ph.D. in communication. Dr. Molitor's detailed analysis of the issue was published in *Health Communication* magazine.

In addition to distorting the actual findings of the research report, aspirin makers have also failed to mention the many negative side effects and dangers presented by taking aspirin.

For instance, they have not explained that:

➤ 1,600 children die each year from allergic reactions to aspirin;

➤ patients with blockage of arteries to the brain are three times more likely to have a stroke if they are taking aspirin;

➤ dyspepsia and gastrointestinal hemorrhage occur in 31% of those taking 300 mgs. of aspirin per day;

➤ even low doses of aspirin can increase the risk of brain hemorrhage; and

➤ that other side effects can include anemia, bleeding ulcers, confusion and dizziness and numerous other problems.

Since they have managed to entice Americans into taking some 25 million aspirin tablets *each day*, the drug manufacturers have no reason to tell the truth ... and every reason to want to perpetuate the lie that aspirin is actually a "health food."

SOURCES: "FDA warns aspirin makers." *Science News,* March 12, 1988 v133 n11 p165(1).

"The preliminary report of the findings of the aspirin component of the ongoing Physicians' Health Study; the FDA perspective on aspirin for the primary prevention of myocardial infarction." *The Journal of the American Medical Association,* June 3, 1988 v259 n21 p3158(3).

"Don't jump the gun with aspirin; there are surer ways to help prevent (heart attacks), ones that don't increase stroke risk," *Medical World News,* May 23, 1988 v29 n10 p50(1).

"High-risk pain pills: though their use is regulated, many common pain remedies can be dangerous, particularly if combined with alcohol or other drugs," *The Atlantic,* Dec. 1989 v264 n6 p36(5).

"Bad Medicine," by William Campbell Douglass, M.D., Second Opinion Publishing, 1995.

"Medicine: What Works & What Doesn't," The Wallace Press, 1995.

Another black mark for aspirin

Aspirin manufacturers have long tried to promote the drug as a safe way to "treat" headaches and other pain. Then, in an effort to boost sales even more, they tried to convince the public that regular doses could actually prevent serious health problems such as cancer, heart attacks and stroke.

A research study, conducted by Dr. Meir J. Stampfer of Brigham and Women's Hospital in Boston, has proven at least one of those assertions false.

One of the myths about aspirin — first put forth in 1994 — was that long-term use of large doses could reduce the risk of breast cancer in women. Dr. Stampfer decided to put that myth to the test. "It was a bit of a long shot," he admitted. "I would have been thrilled if there had been some protection."

The research project — which involved 89,528 female nurses — showed absolutely NO reduction in the breast cancer risk despite the aspirin use.

The report did not indicate if there were any adverse side effects experienced by the women taking the drug. In other research studies, aspirin has consistently been linked to ulcers and other gastrointestinal complications.

SOURCE: "Prospective Study of Regular Aspirin Use and the Risk of Breast Cancer," by Kathleen M. Egan, Meir J. Stampfer, et.al. *Journal of the National Cancer Institute,* July 17, 1996.

Coating doesn't make aspirin safer

By now, most health care consumers know that aspirin increases the risk of bleeding from the upper gastrointestinal (GI) tract. But many of them still believe that coated aspirin is safer.

The pharmaceutical industry has exploited this belief by charging much more for coated aspirin — giving the impression that it's a better product. However, a study published in *The Lancet* shows that coated or buffered aspirin is just as likely as plain aspirin to cause upper GI bleeding.

Aspirin tablets can be coated with cellulose, silicon, or other inactive ingredients (enteric coating) or mixed with buffering agents such as calcium carbonate (chalk).

Dr. Judith Kelly of the Slone Epidemiology Unit, School of Public Health, Boston University School of Medicine, and her colleagues investigated whether these products were less likely to cause upper GI bleeding by asking 550 patients who had an episode of upper GI bleeding and 1,202 healthy participants about their use of aspirin.

The researchers found that taking aspirin — plain, enteric-coated, or buffered — increased the risk of upper GI bleeding about three-fold. At doses above 325 mg., the risk increased about six-fold for plain aspirin and seven-fold for buffered aspirin (there were not enough data to measure the risk associated with enteric-coated aspirin at this higher dose).

Kelly and colleagues concluded that "the assumption that these formulations [enteric-coated and buffered aspirin] are less harmful than plain aspirin may be mistaken."

In a "Commentary" published in the same issue, Dr. Deborah Symmons pointed out that the cost of 75 mg. of enteric-coated aspirin is more than 20 times that of the same dose of plain aspirin.

SOURCE: The Lancet, November 23, 1996.

News about Tylenol risks makes it a hard pill to swallow

By now, most health-conscious Americans know the risks of taking aspirin. Numerous medical research reports have shown that aspirin can cause a wide variety of dangerous side effects, including anemia, bleeding ulcers, confusion, dizziness, dyspepsia, gastrointestinal bleeding, fatal hemorrhages, allergic reactions, increased risk of stroke and brain hemorrhage.

So, they're looking for an alternative. Next to the aspirin bottles on the drug store shelf is a staggering number of other pain pills, but all have their own dangers — including the non- aspirin headache drugs, like Tylenol, which contain acetaminophen.

Tylenol and similar acetaminophen drugs have been linked to both kidney and liver failure.

In January 1996, the *Associated Press* released information about a Johns Hopkins University study which concluded that people who take acetaminophen every day for a year increased their risk of kidney failure by about forty percent. Many newspapers and magazines — which often rely heavily on income from drug manufacturers' ads — did not include the *AP* report.

In March of that year, Tylenol was linked to liver failure. This time, the story was published in *The Washington Times,* but only because a victim paid for a full-page advertisement to get the information to the public.

In the ad, Antonio Benedi tried to refute claims by Tylenol maker McNeil-PPC that its drug was the safest type of pain reliever available on the market.

Not so, Benedi said emphatically! According to the open letter he published as his ad, in 1994, he nearly died after taking the recommended dose of Tylenol for flu symptoms and survived only by an emergency liver transplant. He noted that, although he was in the habit of drinking two to three glasses of wine each night, he abstained from alcohol while he was sick and taking the pills.

He sued McNeil-PPC and won $7.855 million in compensatory damages and an additional $1 million in punitive damages. The verdict was upheld by the U.S. Court of Appeals for the Fourth Circuit, and Benedi used part of the money he received from the case to pay for the *Times* ad.

During the court case, several damaging pieces of evidence came to light. First of all, the link between liver damage and acetaminophen was first reported *three decades ago.*

According to *HealthFacts,* "By the 1980s, the risks of combining alcohol and acetaminophen were well known, and alcoholics were warned away from taking even low doses of acetaminophen."

McNeil-PPC knew of these risks, too.

Court evidence included a company memorandum dated 1986 which clearly instructed sales personnel **not** to discuss with doctors the risk of mixing alcohol and Tylenol.

There was also evidence in McNeil-PPC's own records that 16 deaths had resulted from acetaminophen in combination with alcohol — and they knew about it but never warned people of the risk.

Ironically, Whitehall-Robins Healthcare, maker of the competing pain pill Advil, paid to have Benedi's ad published a few days later in *The New York Times.* They did not add a notice that their own drug — containing ibuprophen — has also been associated with gastrointestinal bleeding and other side effects.

Patients have died, suffered liver failure, been lied to and put at tremendous risk. McNeil- PPC has covered up the facts and deliberately engaged in false advertising. Yet, when the truth was finally uncovered, their only response was to reluctantly put a mild warning on the package, saying people who drink three or more drinks daily should talk to their doctors before using Tylenol.

SOURCES:"Unusual consumer alert about rare risk of Tylenol — drug labeling an issue," HealthFacts, April 1996 v21 n203 p3(2).

Associated Press, January 5, 1996.

Tylenol maker pays $2 million for deceiving public

Nearly 40 million Americans are affected by arthritis so, it's not surprising they search for ways to eliminate their pain.

That's why many of them were optimistic when the McNeil Consumer Products division of drug maker Johnson & Johnson announced its "new" arthritis fighter — an over-the-counter drug so effective that the Arthritis Foundation was endorsing it.

In fact, according to a TV commercial featuring Julie Andrews, the Foundation had "helped to create new *Arthritis Foundation Pain Reliever,* for pain relief we can count on."

What miracle drug did the Arthritis Foundation help create? What revolutionary pain reliever was McNeil offering to arthritis suffers around the country?

The answer: the same old stuff that has filled drug store shelves for years — aspirin, acetaminophen and ibuprofen. The same ingredients you can find in dozens of other "remedies" including *Advil, Excedrin* and Johnson & Johnson-manufactured *Tylenol.*

The only thing "new" about this particular drug was that the Arthritis Foundation was being paid a million dollars for the use of its name.

Not all consumers were fooled.

Retiree Henry Tymecki of Essex Junction, Vermont read the ingredients and realized the entire advertising campaign was bogus. He filed a complaint with his state Attorney General, who started working with AGs from 19 other states to gather information and investigate similar complaints.

McNeil dropped the drug, claiming the decision was based on poor sales, not on the controversy over the misleading advertisements. But the states wanted to pursue the complaints and it appeared that a lengthy legal battle would be causing a new set of headaches for the drug maker.

To avoid that prospect, McNeil chose to settle the dispute out of court, agreeing to pay $250,000 for arthritis research and $90,000 to each of the 19 states to cover legal expenses.

Not surprisingly, both McNeil and the Arthritis Foundation refused to admit any wrongdoing and insisted that the ads offered "an accurate portrayal of these products and their appropriate use in the treatment of arthritis," according to the Arthritis Foundation.

"McNeil decided to settle so as not to incur an expensive legal battle over products that are no longer on the market and we concurred," said Don L. Riggin, president of the Foundation.

In addition, McNeil refunded the purchase price to consumers who sent in a sales receipt or signed statement that they made the purchase, along with the price they paid.

SOURCES: "Arthritis Foundation Announces Voluntary Resolution of State Attorneys General Inquiry," Media release, Arthritis Foundation, October 16, 1996.

"$2 million paid to settle deceptive pain-killer claims," by David Gram, Associated Press, October 17, 1996.

Antacids can make digestive problems worse

People who suffer from arthritis are often desperate for something to relieve their pain and stiffness. Although numerous studies have proven again and again that lifestyle changes such as diet and exercise are the most effective "treatments," an estimated 14 million arthritics continue to take high doses of aspirin and other nonsteroidal anti-inflammatory drugs (also known as NSAIDs) to temporarily relieve the symptoms.

But those drugs can cause ulcers and bleeding. In fact, about 15% of arthritics who take these medications end up with ulcers, compared to only one or two percent of the general population.

What do they do when the ulcer starts to hurt? They turn to yet another type of drug — antacids and acid-blockers such as Tagamet, Zantac and Pepcid.

Instead of helping the situation, however, these drugs usually only make it worse.

A research study showed that the acid-blockers can actually cause more severe gastrointestinal complications and people relying on them are **twice as likely to be hospitalized for ulcers** and related problems than those who do not take the drugs.

The use of antacids to "prevent" digestive disorders has long been contested by non-medical health care professionals.

"The idea of taking an antacid for relief of indigestion is not new," stated nutrition expert A.C. Millett. "It does provide relief. But, when we take an antacid, we need to remember that **digestion stops.**"

Drugs like Tagamet and Zantac "stop digestion (of protein especially) because they both stop HCL production," Millett explained. "Was HCL mistakenly put into our digestion process? I don't think so. Antacids interfere with HCL release and can upset body chemistry resulting in other problems. Long term use can lead to very serious conditions."

Millett advised the public, "Let's quit being misled by antacid ads and the idea that we do not need HCL. No matter what the pharmaceutical companies would like us to believe, use of antacids in any form can lead to health degeneration and disease."

SOURCE: Archives of Internal Medicine, July 1996.

"Being misled on antacids," by A.C. Millett. *The Chiropractic Journal,* August 1996.

Laxatives: One of the most abused and overused OTC drugs

It's one of those drugs which just about everyone has taken at one time or another and it's a common sight in medicine cabinets. But while most people consider over-the-counter (OTC) laxatives as a safe and necessary way to "stay regular," many of these drugs actually pose numerous health hazards and can be physically addictive.

According to *Geriatrics* magazine, "Almost all laxatives are obtained without prescription, and in the United States alone more than 700 different products are sold at an annual cost of $400 million."

Actually, the real dollar amount is nearly double that estimate. The pharmaceutical industry publication, *Drug Topics* puts the amount at $720 million!

Since laxative commercials normally show cheerful, healthy people and use words like "safe," "effective," "natural," and "gentle," most consumers have no idea that they can be harmful or even — in some cases — fatal.

While no drug is completely safe, laxatives have more than their share of dangers and more bad news is uncovered every few months.

In May 1997, the Carcinogen Assessment Committee of the Food and Drug Administration (FDA) reported that an ingredient used in Ex-Lax — phenolphthalein — has been linked to cancer. *ALL* of the laboratory rats subjected to high doses of the drug contracted cancer within six months. Tests indicated that a cancer-suppressing gene normally found in all animals (called gene p53) had vanished from the rats. "There was clear evidence of the loss of p53," stated June Dunnick of the Toxicology Program.

Naturally, the makers of Ex-Lax were quick to argue that they've been using the ingredient for more than 90 years and knew of no risk to consumers who follow directions.

Although further testing will be needed to determine what dose may actually cause the gene loss, there are many other well-documented risks.

A research report published in March 1997, discussed the link between laxatives and hypermagnesemia. Many laxatives contain high levels of magnesium which can increase the serum levels of that element, causing this condition. The report explained that "early symptoms include nausea, vomiting, cutaneous flushing and hyporeflexia (lack of reflexes). Progressive hypermagnesemia can cause a loss of cardiovascular, neuromuscular and respiratory function."

The FDA reported: "Laxative containing water-soluble gums or bulking agents have the potential for swelling and blocking the throat or esophagus if they are taken without adequate fluid. Between 1970 and 1992 there were at least 199 cases of esophageal obstruction and eight cases of asphyxia associated with these products or OTC weight-control products containing these ingredients. There were 18 deaths."

In the April 1991 issue of the *FDA Consumer,* William H. Lipshutz, M.D., clinical professor of medicine at the University of Pennsylvania and head of gastroenterology at Pennsylvania Hospital in Philadelphia warned, "frequent or habitual use of laxatives to promote evacuation can lead to addiction and the ultimate destruction of neurological and muscular control of the large intestine."

In fact, the *FDA Consumer* noted, "Prolonged laxative use can also deplete the body of fluids, salts, and essential vitamins and minerals and inhibit the absorption or effectiveness of other drugs. Furthermore, it can cause dizziness, confusion, fatigue, skin irritation, diarrhea, irregular heartbeat, belching, and a range of other side effects, depending on the laxative used."

The *American Druggist* gave an more detailed look at the possible side effects of this drug:

"Among the most common early symptoms of laxative misuse or abuse are dehydration, abdominal cramping, constipation, diarrhea, nausea, vomiting and bloating," the report informed readers. "Regular use of laxatives tends to weaken the muscles in the intestine, making them less able to function properly. A change in laxative use (including discontinuation) can lead to constipation that is worse than it was initially. Excessive use can lead to lazy bowel syndrome, producing diarrhea or real constipation. Laxatives also can interfere with the effectiveness of other medications."

In addition, some laxatives contain large amounts of sodium, which may worsen conditions like high blood pressure or heart disease. The magnesium and potassium contained in some products can build up in the body if kidney disease is present, and the use of laxatives can reduce the effects of other medications being taken.

Another significant danger is unknowingly taking a laxative during an attack of appendicitis, because the action of the drug can cause the appendix to rupture.

The segment of the population most at risk are our senior citizens, including those who are supposed to be receiving professional medical care at hospitals and in nursing homes.

"Constipation is a common complaint among elderly nursing home residents," explained a team of researchers from Brown University. "Clinical staff frequently respond by prescribing laxatives, but in many cases the resident is not truly constipated and laxative therapy is unnecessary. Over time, excessive laxative use can have serious health consequences, including abdominal bloating and cramps, electrolyte disturbances, watery stools, fecal incontinence, and eventually lower bowel dysmotility, which can result in true constipation."

The situation in many hospitals is no better.

Researchers reporting in *Nursing Times* stated, "Institutions can be places of routine and unquestioned practice in the administration of medications. In one mixed ward of psychogeriatric patients constipation was a common problem for which laxatives were routinely given. In this particular ward, many of the patients were receiving up to five different laxatives a day either orally or rectally. Dementia and being bed or chair-bound greatly increased the risk of chronic constipation. Excessive laxative use is another cause of chronic constipation."

The real problem is a complex one, but centers on the misconception that "regularity" means having one or two bowel movements every day and when they aren't regular, a laxative will solve the problem.

"The public should get out of the habit of taking a quick laxative fix," said Dr. Lipshutz. But such common sense advice is quickly drowned out by the blare of television and radio commercials which promise instant, gentle relief without ever mentioning the risks involved.

Unfortunately, the problem may get worse in the next few years, as the drug manufacturing industry steps up its marketing effort.

"The U.S. laxative market, which has been relatively slow-growing of late, is likely to benefit greatly from the aging of the population," Lipshutz added. "As the Baby Boom Generation approaches middle-age, the $720-million category is expected to pick up considerably."

Sadly, so will the side effects and deaths caused by the abuse and overuse of these potentially dangerous products. Since the drug companies cannot be expected to put public welfare ahead of profits — and since the FDA is unwilling to oppose them despite the overwhelming evidence that these drugs are unsafe — it will be up to the consumers to make the healthy, and smart, decisions.

SOURCES: Report presented at a meeting of the Carcinogen Assessment Committee, Food and Drug Administration, May 1997.

"Acute hypermagnesemia after use of laxatives," by Dr. Richard Sadovsky. *American Family Physician, March 1997.*

"A strategy to reduce laxative use among older people," by E. Stewart, et. al., Royal Cornhill Hospital, Aberdeen. Nursing Times, Jan. 22, 1997.

United States Pharmacopeial Convention Inc., 1996.

"Constipation: common-sense care of the older patient," by Drs. Abdul Abyad and Fadi Mourad. Geriatrics, December 1996.

"The misuse and abuse of OTC laxatives," by Ara DerMarderosian and Sharon Brudnicki. American Druggist, Jan. 1996.

"Unnecessary laxative therapy can worsen constipation, decrease quality of life." The Brown University Long-Term Care Quality Letter, July 10, 1995.

"Seniors a key to strong laxative sales." Drug Topics, Feb. 20, 1995.

"New warnings required for OTC antacids, laxatives,"
FDA Consumer, Nov. 1993.

"Constipation is a symptom, not a disease," by Janet Lepke. Environmental Nutrition, June 1993.

"Overuse hazardous: Laxatives rarely needed," by Mike Cummings. FDA Consumer, April 1991.

Ban on OTC sale of laxative ingredient proposed by FDA

The Food & Drug Administration (FDA) has proposed a ban on the over-the-counter (OTC) sale of phenolphthalein, an ingredient widely used in laxatives, because it may pose long-term safety concerns. The proposal would require that products containing this ingredient either be reformulated or withdrawn from the market.

The proposal to reclassify phenolphthalein as unsafe was based on a review of studies carried out under the National Toxicology Program (NTP) and presented at an FDA meeting.

After reviewing the NTP material and other data, the FDA committee concluded that phenolphthalein, which has been used in several products — including *Ex-Lax* — for many years, potentially could cause cancer in humans. Because consumers have access to more than two dozen laxative products without this ingredient, the FDA considered that phenolphthalein's benefits do not outweigh its risks.

Health Watch first alerted its readers to the potential dangers of phenolphthalein in its June 1997 issue. At that time, results of the NTP studies were reported in which *ALL* of the laboratory rats subjected to high doses of the drug contracted cancer within six months. Tests indicated that a cancer-suppressing gene normally found in all animals (called gene p53) had vanished from the rats.

Then, the makers of *Ex-Lax* argued that they'd been using the ingredient for more than 90 years and knew of no risk to consumers who follow directions.

Tragically, there is no way to determine how many people may have died or been afflicted with cancer caused by this or other OTC chemical compounds.

The FDA proposed reclassifying phenolphthalein as a Category II ingredient, or an ingredient not generally recognized as "safe and effective."

*SOURCES:*Food and Drug Administration Media Alert. August 29, 1997.

Report presented at a meeting of the Carcinogen Assessment Committee, Food and Drug Administration, May 1997.

Extensive decongestant use linked to stroke

According to a study released during the American Academy of Neurology's 49th Annual Meeting, extensive use of common over-the-counter (OTC) decongestants contained in some allergy medicines, cough syrup, and other drugs may cause stroke.

Decongestants constrict the blood vessels in and around the nose to eliminate congestion.

"Decongestants can potentially affect blood vessels in both the brain and heart and can elevate blood pressure," said senior author Eric Raps, M.D., director of the Division of Stroke and Neurointensive Care at the University of Pennsylvania Medical Center.

This two-year study looked at five stroke patients under age 60 who were not at high risk for stroke. It revealed that all had been using OTC decongestants for extended periods. Four of the five patients had been taking pseudoephedrine. The study found that the strokes may be related to OTC decongestant vasoconstrictive effects on the brain.

"The study indicated that it may be possible to identify patients who run a higher risk of stroke when using decongestants," stated lead author Lidgia Vives, M.D., stroke and neurointensive care fellow at the University of Pennsylvania Medical Center.

Some individuals whose blood vessels have a tendency to constrict easier than others may be more sensitive to decongestants. Conditions that suggest this tendency include livedo reticularis (a discoloration of the skin bearing a bluish net-like pattern), Raynaud's Phenomenon (a change in the color of the skin triggered by exposure to cold weather), or migraine. People with these conditions may be at a higher risk for stroke when using decongestants.

Pseudoephedrine is found in a wide variety of OTC drugs, including many of the popular cold and flu capsules which the public generally thinks of as "safe." Ironically, the people who usually find this decongestant more effective are the ones at greatest risk.

SOURCE: Media advisory, American Academy of Neurology, April 16, 1997.

OTC eyedrops may take redness out ... but can put pink in

They claim to "take the redness out" of eyes, but over-the-counter eyedrops may cause conjunctivitis, a highly contagious eye disease known as "pink eye."

According to a study published in an opthamology journal, decongestant eyedrops which contain the vasoconstrictors (agents that narrow the blood vessels) *naphazoline, tetrahydrozoline,* or *phenylephrinecan* "produce acute and chronic forms of conjunctivitis by pharmacological, toxic, and allergic mechanisms. Once recognized, conjunctival inflammation often takes several weeks to resolve."

Conjunctivitis is characterized by inflammation, redness, discomfort and discharge.

SOURCE: *Archives of Ophthalmology,* Jan. 1997.

Drug labels not telling the whole story

Many prescription and over-the-counter drugs contain ingredients which can cause seizures, headaches, bronchospasm and diarrhea. Yet, as serious as these side effects are, the ingredients are not listed on the bottle!

Since they are considered "inactive" ingredients, drug companies can put a wide variety of sweeteners, dyes, coloring agents and preservatives into their drugs and not list them on the packages.

The FDA has approved nearly 800 of these chemicals, even though almost all of them can cause negative side effects in some people.

The problem is particularly serious when it comes to drugs made for and marketed to children, who are often more sensitive to these chemicals.

According to a survey of labels on 102 chewable and liquid pediatric pharmaceuticals, 90% contained sweeteners, 80% contained dyes and coloring agents and 65% contained preservatives. But most did not detail which sweeteners, dyes or preservatives were used.

Listing the specific ingredients is voluntary, and manufacturers can avoid listing them by saying they are protecting their "trade secrets."

Ironically, when the FDA proposed major drug labeling changes, it made no mention of listing inactive ingredients, even those which might pose health risks to consumers. Instead, the main provision of the proposed regulation merely involves a new label format, going so far as to specify a "bulleted, easier-to-read format," and minimum type sizes and styles.

SOURCES: Pediatrics, February 1997.

"FDA proposes new, easy to understand labeling for OTC drugs," FDA press announcement, Feb. 26, 1997.

Common pain reliever can cause liver damage

High doses of acetaminophen — the primary ingredient in many over-the-counter pain relievers — caused liver injury in some patients, reported researchers at the UT Southwestern Medical Center at Dallas. The risk is particularly high when mixed with alcohol.

Dr. William Lee, professor of internal medicine, and his team of liver-disease researchers reviewed the records of 589 patients who were treated at Dallas County's Parkland Memorial Hospital from 1992 to 1995.

From that group he found 71 patients who were hospitalized with liver damage after taking acetaminophen, the most common cause of acute liver failure.

"Our study suggests we should be more diligent in educating the public and physicians about the risks associated with acetaminophen because it's commonplace for people to reach for a bottle of pain reliever without thinking about possible complications," said Dr. Lee, who directs the Liver Diseases Clinical Center at UT Southwestern's James W. Aston Ambulatory Care Center.

Lee speculated that acetaminophen causes liver damage in alcoholic or fasting patients because alcohol and fasting deplete the body of glutathione, a detoxification agent normally found in large quantities in the liver.

He cautioned that even people who aren't alcoholics but who consume alcohol before or after taking acetaminophen can experience liver damage.

SOURCE: The New England Journal of Medicine, October 15, 1997.

Chapter 13

Testing, testing...

Diagnostic testing has become the new darling of the medical profession. Often, these expensive tests are merely the M.D.'s way of avoiding potential malpractice suits, but just as often they are easy ways to pad a patient's bill.

Which tests are really needed? Which are just scams or — at best — the result of ignorance and fear of liability? That's a difficult question for most patients to answer since the medical profession is reluctant to look closely at the problem and provide accurate advice. On the rare occasion when a medical panel or agency issues a report stating that certain tests are unnecessary, the outrage from profit-motivated trade organizations like the American Medical Association quickly silences the opposition.

Many medical tests unnecessary, University researchers say

One of the major reasons why the cost of American health care is skyrocketing is that doctors are performing numerous tests on patients — including many which are not only unnecessary but can actually be risky.

A University of Michigan physician and three co-authors explored this problem in an article in the *Archives of Family Medicine.* The lead researcher was David J. Doukas, M.D., associate professor in the U-M Department of Family Medicine and associate director for clinical bioethics in the U-M Program in Society and Medicine.

The article described several potential risks of screening tests with controversial benefits, including:

— Reliance on screening tests before their effectiveness has been corroborated by adequate research.

— Creating the impression that such exams can reduce a patient's risk to zero, possibly leading them to make uninformed medical decisions.

— Inaccurate, false positive results which can cause profound anxiety and require additional testing that can be increasingly invasive and costly.

— Depleting society's limited medical resources.

Doukas and his colleagues pointed out, for instance, that there is considerable disagreement in the medical community over the routine use of mammograms in women under the age of 50 and prostate specific antigen tests in men.

Yet, these tests have helped produce multi- billion dollar industries in recent years.

The researchers claimed that doctors often provide controversial screening tests because they fear a future lawsuit by a patient who later develops a disease.

In addition, patients frequently request a test because they read an article about it in a magazine, or found out that their insurance company will pay for it.

Rather than educate patients about the risks involved, many doctors simply give the tests upon demand — and charge patients for them.

The article noted that physicians have a responsibility to inform patients of the limitations and risks of screening tests — and to refuse to order tests that would violate their medical and ethical judgment. Physicians can counsel patients about the lack of scientific evidence regarding a test's benefits and the fact that no test can assure zero-risk of disease.

This education and negotiation process is intended to make the patient aware of which screening tests have been proven to be beneficial and which have not. Such a discussion can result in patients making informed and learned health care decisions.

"For most diseases for which there is a potential screening test, the effectiveness of screening is controversial," the article stated. "Physicians can use a 'preventive ethics' approach to explain that tests with controversial benefits are unlikely to be helpful."

SOURCE: "Ethical Considerations in the Provision of Controversial Screening Tests," *Archives of Family Practice,* Oct. 17, 1997.

No evidence that men over 50 need prostate screening

Not long ago, a panel of experts at the National Institutes of Health Consensus Development Conference declared that there is no proof that the potential benefits of mammograms outweigh the risks involved for women under 50 years of age.

A number of "cancer societies" argued, saying the tests (which range in cost between $50 and $200 each) are a necessity for all women over 40 — despite the fact that radiation from yearly mammograms during ages 40-49 has been estimated to cause one additional breast cancer death per 10,000 women.

A study by the Prostate Disease Patient Outcomes Research Team (PORT) stated that men over 50 probably don't benefit from prostate screening. Not surprisingly, those same cancer societies — which are run by and for medical doctors and pharmaceutical companies — are disputing *that* conclusion.

According to the PORT, which is supported by the U.S. Government's Agency for Health Care Policy and Research (AHCPR), there is insufficient evidence to support performing an annual digital rectal examination and prostate-specific antigen (PSA) screening on men over 50 years of age as recommended by the American Cancer Society.

Using data from large studies, the PORT constructed a model to estimate the risks, maximum benefits, and cost-effectiveness of a one-time screening in a hypothetical group of 100,000 men in their 50s, 60s, and 70s, using both digital rectal exams and PSA tests.

Out of this 100,000 men, the researchers estimated that the recommended screening would result in as many as 27,000 biopsies of the prostate each year, cause up to 23 surgical deaths, make nearly 1,600 men impotent, more than 300 incontinent and 500 both impotent and incontinent.

Even when their model assumed effective treatment following confirmed local prostate cancer, screening added just six days to two-and-a-half weeks to the average life expectancy of older men.

"The lack of direct evidence showing a net benefit of screening for prostate cancer mandates more clinician-patient discussion for this procedure than for many other routine tests," concluded team leader, Michael J. Barry, M.D., of Harvard Medical School.

SOURCE: "Early detection of prostate cancer: Part I: Prior probability and effectiveness of tests," and "Early detection of prostate cancer: Part II: Estimating the risks, benefits, and costs," by Christopher M. Coley, M.D., et al, *Annals of Internal Medicine,* March 1 & 15, 1997.

Chapter 14

Just "female" troubles

W omen have long been the victim of a male dominated medical system and, even today, they are treated more as a potential "market" than as patients. Although Dr. Robert Mendelsohn exposed the shameful way medicine treats women in his 1981 book, "MalePractice," things haven't changed all that much. It remains all too true, as Dr. Mendelsohn said, that "If you are a woman living in America, the greatest danger to your health is, in all likelihood, your own doctor."

This is all too evident in the burgeoning "menopause" industry. Although women have been going through the same hormonal cycle for a million years — a cycle which is perfectly normal and natural — the medical profession has suddenly classified the change of life as a disease requiring medical treatment. In trying to improve on the natural design of a women's system, they have bombarded her with artificial drugs which disrupt the normal cycle and pose significant dangers to her general health. Yet they seldom ask why women in so many other countries do not suffer from the symptoms which the medications are supposed to relieve. If they did, they would find that diet and lifestyle alone could make this life passage nearly pain- and discomfort-free — without the risk of drugs.

Link between hormone replacement therapy and breast cancer increase suggested

Current use of hormone replacement therapy (HRT) might increase the risk of breast cancer detected between routine mammographic screens.

That's the conclusion voiced by Dr. Valerie Beral and colleagues in a letter published in the correspondence section of the British medical journal, *The Lancet*.

An earlier report in *Lancet* showed an increase in interval cancers of the breast — those which develop between mammographic screens — and that the rise was higher in women aged 50-59 years than in those aged 60-64. The breast cancers arose in women who had had a previous negative result. In the United Kingdom, screening is undertaken three every years in women over 50, so these cancers had developed in the three years between mammographic examinations.

Because the rate of interval cancers was higher in the younger age group studied in this report, Beral and co-workers suggested that the increase is due to HRT use — women aged 50-59 being more likely to be under such treatment than women in the older age group.

The authors pointed to the only study that has looked at interval cancers in relation to HRT use. That investigation suggested that the use of HRT reduced the chances of cancer being detected by mammography, probably because this treatment increases the mammographic density of the breast — as natural oestrogen (hormone produced by the ovaries) does in younger women.

More and more women are using HRT, and how much this hormone treatment contributes to the high rate of interval cancers seen in the UK breast screening program needs to be established, according to Beral and coauthors.

"The available evidence is too uncertain to guide policy," said the doctors, but they suggested that "women stop using hormone replacement therapy for a short period before being screened."

SOURCES: Is the increase in breast cancer between mammographic screens due to hormone replacement therapy? (Correspondence), by Dr. Valerie Beral. *The Lancet,* April 12, 1997.

Hormone replacement therapy and high incidence of breast cancer between mammographic screens," *The Lancet* Feb. 15, 1997.

More bad news for estrogen therapy

In recent years, the medical profession has successfully portrayed menopause as a *disease,* one which can be treated by artificially boosting the level of estrogen in women — even though that "change" is a natural part of female development.

This erroneous assessment has allowed estrogen replacement therapy (ERT) to become a multi-billion dollar industry luring millions of healthy women into doctors' offices each year.

But ERT also has serious risks, according to several research reports.

The most serious drawback is that women who subject themselves to ERT may be more than twice as likely to get breast cancer than women who do not take the hormone.

An article in *The Journal of the American Medical Association (JAMA)* reported that estrogen increases bone mineral density (BMD), which in turn is linked to the higher incidence of breast cancer.

Jane A. Cauley, Dr.PH., from the Department of Epidemiology, University of Pittsburgh, Pa., and colleagues studied 6,854 women and found that the age-adjusted incidence rate of breast cancer was lowest among those with low BMD. Women with the highest BMD had two to two-and-a-half times increased risk of breast cancer compared with those with the lowest BMD.

The researchers stated, "Our findings suggest that before estrogen replacement therapy becomes widely used for indications other than osteoporosis, that the balance of risks and benefits of hormone replacement therapy should be reevaluated with respect to BMD, osteoporosis, breast cancer, and coronary heart disease."

An earlier report by the *Journal of the National Cancer Institute* found that an increase in breast density caused by ERT can look like a tumor during a mammography test and lead to a false positive test result. The "false alarms" could "increase the cost of breast cancer screening and ... may decrease its effectiveness," the report concluded.

As if all that weren't bad enough, ERT has also proven to be less effective in preventing osteoporosis and heart disease than a change in diet. In fact, the *American Journal of Clinical Nutrition* published a report which showed that eliminating meat from the diet can cut urinary calcium losses in half.

These facts have left many health care professionals wondering why M.D.s are still so quick to prescribe ERT. Many medical experts say that the doctors are only responding to the demands of their patients who want to be able to eat whatever they want and take a pill for what ails them.

"That's nonsense," said the Physicians Committee on Responsible Medicine (PCRM) in a June 20, 1996 report. "It is patronizing to assume that every postmenopausal woman is too wedded to her current diet and lifestyle to listen to competent advice. The real problem is, she is not likely to find such advice.

"Most doctors know little about how diet affects health," continued PCRM, "even when a mountain of research has already been done, and is gathering dust in medical libraries. They rely instead on knee-jerk prescribing, which is continually encouraged by drug manufacturers' aggressive promotions."

The PCRM report concluded: "When doctors learn how to use all the tools their medical bags could really offer — including prescriptions for diet and lifestyle changes — their patients will be much better off."

SOURCES:"Urinary calcium, sodium, and bone mass of young females," *American Journal of Clinical Nutrition,* August 1995 v62 n2 p417(9).

"Effect of estrogen replacement therapy on the specificity and sensitivity of screening mammography," by Mary B. Laya, et. al. *Journal of the National Cancer Institute,* May 15, 1996.

"Estrogen Dangers Before and After Menopause," Physicians' Committee for Responsible Medicine (PCRM), June 20, 1996.

"Effects of Hormone Therapy on Bone Mineral Density, Results From the Postmenopausal Estrogen/Progestin Interventions (PEPI) Trial," *Journal of the American Medical Association,* Nov. 6, 1996.

"High bone mineral density can double the risk of breast cancer," media advisory, American Medical Association, Nov. 6, 1996.

Hormone replacement therapy — no protection for heart disease

The belief that hormone replacement therapy (HRT) for postmenopausal women may protect against cardiovascular disease is based on inadequate evidence, said researchers in the *British Medical Journal.*

Researchers from Finland and the United Kingdom studied the results of 22 trials involving 4,124 women and found no evidence that short term use of HRT protected against heart disease.

Since results of long term trials will not be available for some time, there's no way to determine the long-term effects for either cancer or cardiovascular disease, the study's authors added.

There have been hundreds of trials studying the impact of HRT, but adverse effects have not been systematically reported, said the authors.

The medical profession has pushed HRT on women for several years, often claiming it can prevent heart disease or cancer despite evidence that it can have severe and possibly deadly side effects. However, few doctors have received proper training about the therapy and many rely on drug company representatives for most of their information.

In a Gallup poll, 80% of the physicians responding said they discuss hormone replacement therapy with their female patients, but only 45% said they had extensive medical training in the use of HRT in menopausal and post-menopausal women.

SOURCE: *British Medical Journal*, No 7101 Volume 315, 19 July 1997.

"Safer" hormone replacement drug can actually double risk of cancer

For years, the medical profession has been trying to convince women that their natural menopause cycle is actually a disease which has to be "treated" with potent drugs.

Those who buy into this medical myth may end up taking estrogen "replacement" drugs, which can make them twice as likely to get breast cancer than women who do not take the hormone. The estrogen increases bone mineral density, which in turn is linked to the higher incidence of breast cancer.

That was the conclusion of a research study published in *The Journal of the American Medical Association.*

To offset that side effect, women are also given a second hormone, progestin. However, a study published in the *Journal of the National Cancer Institute* stated progestin can cause double the risk of cancer of the uterine lining. To avoid this risk, researchers say, women must stay on the drug for at least 14 days out of every month.

"The only other large study to look at this cyclic therapy showed there was still a bit of an increased risk, 2.5- or 3-fold increased risk, even if you used it for 10 days per month," stated Dr. Deborah Grady, an associate professor of epidemiology and medicine at the University of California, San Francisco.

In a patronizing statement that appears to underestimate women's intelligence, Dr. Deborah Grady commented: "That's what leads us to recommend 14 days — it's a nice round number that women can remember."

Progestin can also cause side effects such as depression, menstrual-like bleeding, or spotting.

SOURCES: *Journal of the National Cancer Institute* (1997;89:1110-1116).

"Effects of Hormone Therapy on Bone Mineral Density, Results From the Postmenopausal Estrogen/Progestin Interventions (PEPI) Trial," *Journal of the American Medical Association,* Nov. 6, 1996.

"High bone mineral density can double the risk of breast cancer," media advisory, American Medical Association, Nov. 6, 1996.

Common biopsy technique ineffective

A technique commonly used to detect breast cancer often doesn't work. That was the conclusion of a medical research project conducted by the Radiologic Diagnostic Oncology Group. According to the study, fine needle aspiration biopsies frequently do not collect enough breast tissue to make any diagnosis.

Fine needle aspiration biopsies use a very small needle to remove tissue from the area of the breast that appears abnormal on the mammogram. The needle can be inserted into the tissue guided by mammography (stereotactically) or by ultrasound.

An analysis of 351 women who had fine needle aspiration biopsies revealed that, overall, more than a third of the biopsies provided an insufficient tissue sample, stated Dr. Etta Pisano, associate professor of radiology at the University of North Carolina-Chapel Hill and chair of the study. The insufficient sample rate was even higher for some breast abnormalities.

Dr. Pisano presented the study at the American College of Radiology's (ACR's) "27th National Conference on Breast Cancer" in Dallas on April 30, 1996.

SOURCE: "Study Criticizes Fine Needle Biopsy Test for Breast Cancer." News release by the American College of Radiology, April 30, 1996.

Experts fail to agree on need for under-50 mammograms

Until recently, the medical community appeared united in its support of mammograms as a way to save women's lives by giving them early warning of breast cancer.

And, at $50-200 a test, mammograms have become a cash cow for many doctors and radiologists, particularly since many medical agencies have encouraged women as young as 40 years old to receive the tests.

Now, however, the medical community is divided because of a serious disagreement about the wisdom of subjecting women under the age of 50 to these tests.

According to a panel of experts who gathered for the National Institutes of Health (NIH) Consensus Development Conference in January 1997, there is no proof that the potential benefits of mammograms outweigh the risks involved for this age group.

In refusing to recommend the test for women under 50, the panel pointed out that breast cancer is relatively rare in women under 50 and that there is only a 0.3% chance of dying from the disease during this decade of their lives.

Although various medical organizations often claim that research has shown mammograms are responsible for saving and extending lives, the panel disagreed. "The information from the RCTs (randomized controlled trials) also allows an estimate of no lives extended for 1,000 women regularly screened from ages 40 to 49," the panel noted.

Of course, if the mammogram was without risk, the test might be considered nothing more than yet another unnecessary medical examination (although an expensive one). But the mammogram is not risk-free and the NIH panel experts found that the risks do NOT outweigh the very small possible benefit for a few women.

According to the draft report of the panel, "An understanding of the nature and magnitude of risks is important to both primary care providers and women making informed decisions about breast cancer screening." Some of the potential risks they listed were:

➤ *Risks associated with false-negative examinations.* "Up to one-fourth of all invasive breast cancers are not detected by mammography in 40 to 49 year olds, compared with one-tenth of cancers in 50 to 59 year olds," the report stated.

➤ *Additional diagnostic testing induced by false-positive examinations.* "Many mammographic abnormalities may not be due to cancer, but will prompt additional testing and anxiety," the panel found. In a Swedish study of 60,000 women aged 40-64, 726 were referred to oncologists for treatment for cancer — *but 70% of them were actually found to be cancer free!* Some 86% of women under 50 who were referred for cancer treatment had actually triggered a false positive test result.

On average, every woman whose mammogram results in an "abnormal," reading is subjected to two additional diagnostic tests (e.g., diagnostic mammography, ultrasound, needle aspiration, core biopsy, or surgical biopsy), according to the NIH panel.

Compounding the problem with false positive results is the fact that estrogen therapy increases the likelihood of a false positive result by seventy-one percent!

➤ *Psychosocial consequences.* "There is concern that women having abnormal mammograms — both true positive and false-positive — experience psychosocial sequelae, including inconvenience, anxiety, and fear."

➤ *Radiation exposure.* "The risk of radiation-induced breast cancer has long been a concern to mammographers and has driven the efforts to minimize radiation dose per examination," the panel explained. "Radiation can cause breast cancer in women, and the risk is proportional to dose. The younger the woman at the time of exposure, the greater her lifetime risk for breast cancer.

"Radiation-related breast cancers occur at least 10 years after exposure," continued the panel. "Radiation from yearly mammograms during ages 40-49 has been estimated to cause one additional breast cancer death per 10,000 women."

Other medical research has shown that the incidence of a form of breast cancer known as ductal carcinoma *in situ* (DCIS), which accounts for 12% of all breast cancer cases, increased by 328% — and 200% of this increase is due to the use of mammography!

After examining the risks from mammograms as well as the potential benefits, the panel concluded: "At the present time, the available data do not warrant a single recommendation for mammography for all women in their forties."

The NIH panel conclusions echoed the decision made by the National Cancer Institute several years ago when it chose not to recommend mammograms to women under the age of 50. However, numerous other cancer groups — including the American Cancer Society and the American College of Radiology — continue to encourage young women to undergo the risky tests.

SOURCES: *British Medical Journal,* February 1996.

The Journal of the American Medical Association, March 27, 1996.

National Institutes of Health Consensus Development Statement (draft), "Breast Cancer Screening for Women Ages 40-49," Jan. 21-23, 1997.

"The financial politics of mammograms," *Alternative Medicine Digest,* Issue 15, Jan./Feb. 1997.

Most M.D.s unaware of differences in heart disease in men and women

Results from a national Gallup survey found nearly two-thirds of the nation's primary care physicians inaccurately reported "no difference" in the symptoms, warning signs and diagnosis of heart disease in women, compared to men.

The survey, commissioned by Washington Hospital Center, asked 256 internists and family practitioners across the country to determine medical doctors' awareness of the prevalence, severity and signs of heart disease in women.

"If a physician follows the classic male model for diagnosing heart disease, a huge number of women with heart disease will be missed," said Washington Hospital Center cardiologist Patricia Davidson, M.D. "Both women and their physicians must be aware that the symptoms of women's heart disease are different from men's."

Heart disease is the leading cause of death among American women, each year claiming 233,000 lives — six times the number of women who die of breast cancer annually.

Prevalence of the disease among women is also high. Each year, 625,000 women suffer a heart attack. Over 28 million American women are living with the effects of cardiovascular disease, including heart disease, high blood pressure and stroke. Of these, more than one-half are under the age of 65.

While angina (chest pain) is a major indicator of heart disease in both women and men, other symptoms in women, such as shortness of breath and chronic fatigue, are very common and are often being ignored.

Although two-out-of-three physicians surveyed identified shortness of breath as a warning sign of heart disease in women, chronic fatigue was listed by fewer than one-out-of-five respondents and only 10% mentioned other important symptoms for women, including nausea, dizziness or swelling of the ankles.

In addition, the Gallup survey found that:

➤ Only 39% of the doctors had extensive medical training in diagnosing heart disease in women, compared to 69% who said they had extensive training in diagnosing the same disease in men.

➤ 68% said there is no difference in diagnostic tests for men and women, when in actuality heart disease can be diagnosed more effectively and accurately in women using a nuclear stress test or stress echocardiogram, rather than a simple treadmill electrocardiogram (ECG), commonly called a stress test.

➤ Half of those surveyed listed a health problem other than heart disease as the greatest health risk facing women over 50. Breast cancer was listed by 18% and 10% said osteoporosis. Yet, twice as many women die of cardiovascular disease each year than die of all forms of cancer combined.

SOURCE: "Majority of primary care physicians unaware of differences in heart disease in men and women; many cases of heart disease in women undiagnosed," Center for Cardiovascular Education, Nov. 21, 1996.

M.D.s fail to diagnose sleep apnea in women

When men complain of daytime sleepiness and snoring, doctors take them seriously and think of the possibility of sleep apnea, a serious and potentially fatal disorder. However, when women patients complain of identical symptoms, they are often dismissed as "women's problems" or emotional problems such as depression.

That was the conclusion of a University of Wisconsin (UW) Medical School study published in the *Archives of Internal Medicine.* The study showed that women with sleep apnea have the same standard symptoms as men do — but that many more men are diagnosed with the disorder than women.

"Health care providers may not be asking the right follow-up questions or prescribing additional tests when women come to them with these symptoms, which are automatically associated with sleep apnea in men," said UW Medical School professor of preventive medicine Terry Young, Ph.D. "This may explain why sleep disorder clinics are filled predominantly with men, even though we have found that at least a quarter of the people with sleep apnea are women."

Sleep apnea consists of episodes of breathing pauses during sleep that may lead to other health problems, including hypertension.

In 1993, Young reported in the *New England Journal of Medicine* that many more women than previously suspected experience breathing disorders related to sleep apnea. She and her colleagues noted a male-to-female ratio of three-to-one, much different than the ten-to-one ratio usually seen in sleep clinics.

The observation came from the Sleep Cohort Study, an on-going population-based investigation of cardiopulmonary problems linked to sleep disorders. Approximately 1,200 randomly selected Wisconsin state employees have been studied so far in an overnight stay at the General Clinical Research Center of the University of Wisconsin Hospital and Clinics.

In the study, the UW researchers sought to learn if fewer women were diagnosed with sleep apnea because they had different symptoms than men. Participants consisted of 551 men and 388 women between the ages of 30 and 60 randomly selected for an overnight study.

"We hypothesized three possible explanations for the gender disparity in sleep apnea diagnosis," said Young. "Women could be embarrassed to report they snore, they might have different symptoms than men, or doctors might not link sleep apnea in women to snoring and daytime sleepiness, as they do with men."

The study revealed that women with various levels of sleep apnea did not experience symptoms that differed significantly from those in men with the same apnea levels. What's more, women showed no reluctance to admit they snored.

"The most viable explanation for the disparity is that health care providers are not taking women seriously when they complain of these symptoms," said Young. "This may be true particularly when women report psychological problems such as depression at the same time as they describe sleepiness and snoring."

SOURCES: *Annuals of Internal Medicine,* Dec. 1996.
Media advisory, University of Wisconsin, Dec. 12, 1996.

Nurse-midwives a better option for most pregnant women

Many hospitals subject pregnant women to unnecessary hi-tech medical intervention when they give birth, and ignore the benefits offered by certified nurse-midwives (CNMs), according to an article in the medical journal *Public Health Reports,* an official publication of the United States Public Health Service.

The article, "The Beneficial Alternative: Nurse-Midwifery," reported that although most pregnancies and births do not require medical intervention, certain obstetric procedures like ultrasonography and electronic fetal monitoring are used in most deliveries directed by physicians.

Women who have their babies without CNMs are also more likely to be denied room to walk around during labor to ease their discomfort, more likely to be denied the use of a bath or shower during their labor, and more likely to undergo unnecessary cesarean surgery.

"Instead of a last-minute rush to deploy all the latest expensive equipment, hospitals should see childbirth for what it is — a normal event," said Dr. Sidney Wolfe, Director of Public Citizen's Health Research Group and co-author of the article with Mary Gabay. "Nurse- midwives provide more individualized care, and they reduce the rate of expensive medical interventions."

Although the preference for in-hospital midwife-attended births in the U.S. is growing (up from 19,686 in 1975 to 196,977 in 1994), only about five percent of births in the U.S. happen in this way. In Europe, midwives are the principal attendants for more than 75% of births. The U.S. also has a relatively high infant mortality rate. In 1994, it ranked 21st among other major developed countries.

"For most pregnant women, certified nurse-midwives offer a better alternative than physicians," stated Dr. Wolfe. "Certified nurse-midwives offer the sort of care not provided by many hospitals." The article showed that nurse-midwifery care results in outcomes similar to those achieved by physicians, often at much lower cost.

In a "opposing viewpoint" article published in the same issue of *Public Health Reports,* Dr. Hal C. Lawrence, an obstetrician and co-chairman of an American College of Obstetricians and Gynecologists Committee, rejected the suggestion that CNMs are often the best option, charging that "collaborative teams of physicians and advance practice professionals" are preferable.

Wolfe vigorously opposed the suggestion that doctors always know best.

"Diminishing the importance of the crucial independent role played by nurse-midwives is insulting to their talent and expertise. Reducing these highly-trained professionals to the role of physicians' handmaidens is outrageous."

The Public Citizen authors analyzed a list of options usually offered by CNMs and compared how many were offered to non-CNM patients (under the care of ob-gyn doctors) at the same hospitals. They found that during labor and delivery, CNM patients were more likely than non-CNM patients to be offered oral fluids, to ambulate during labor, to be encouraged to use alternative positions for delivery and to be allowed friends in attendance at the birth.

"More CNMs should be trained, and the public made aware of their effectiveness. In many states, restrictive regulation hinders CNMs. These restrictions include limitations on hospital admitting privileges, prescribing privileges and lack of mandatory third-party insurance reimbursement," Wolfe pointed out.

Florida, by contrast, is aggressively promoting the use of CNMs as a cost-effective answer to a shortage of maternal health care providers. Florida aims to have 50% of healthy pregnant women cared for by midwives by the year 2000 and aims to train 600 additional nurse- midwives by that year.

"If other states follow Florida's lead, excessive use of costly and needless medical interventions can be cut, and the infant mortality rate greatly improved," said Wolfe.

SOURCE: "The Beneficial Alternatives: Nurse-Midwifery" by the Public Citizen's Health Research Group, *Public Health Reports,* Sept. 1, 1997.

M.D. 'ignorance' blamed in cancer deaths

According to a spokesman for the National Cancer Institute (NCI), the vast majority of surgeons who operate on women for early-stage ovarian cancer do not properly check to see if the disease has spread — and their failure may be causing the unnecessary death of thousands of women.

Ninety percent of women who undergo surgery for early-stage ovarian cancer run the risk of dying from it later because surgeons are ignorant about how ovarian cancer spreads, stated Dr. Edward Trimble of the NCI. He made his remarks during the annual meeting of the American Society for Clinical Oncology, May 18-21, 1996. When the more advanced cancer is not detected, Dr. Trimble said, "her disease recurs, and she dies."

Trimble's statements were based upon a study which showed that only 10% of the 785 women studied, received proper treatment.

SOURCES: "Ovarian cancer: Do doctors know best? 90 percent of women in study get sub-standard treatment," by Medical Correspondent Jeff Levine. CNN Interactive. May 21, 1996.

"Study: Ovarian cancer spread not checked." Associated Press, May 21, 1996.

M.D.s misdiagnose more than half of rapid heart rhythm cases

Frequently, when patients complain of recurrent, rapid heart rhythm, they're told they're just having 'panic attacks' and urged to relax or take tranquilizers. This is particularly true if the patient happens to be a woman.

Timothy J. Lessmeier, M.D., formerly of Wayne State University School of Medicine, and now with Heart Clinics Northwest, Spokane, Washington, and colleagues studied 107 patients who were referred for a special heart catheterization procedure known as electrophysiologic testing. The median age of the patients was 40 and 55% were women.

The test proved the patients were actually experiencing a recurrent, non-life-threatening disorder known as paroxysmal supraventricular tachycardia (PSVT). PSVT causes a rapid heartbeat, typically 150-250 beats per minute, that often stops on its own after several seconds or minutes.

The researchers reported that the disorder was incorrectly diagnosed for 55% of the patients during their initial medical evaluations. Among those unrecognized cases, a median of 3.3 years went by before the correct diagnosis was made.

They stated that in more than half of the unrecognized cases, the initial physicians attributed symptoms to panic, anxiety or stress. The misdiagnosis was made twice as frequently for women as for men. Twelve percent of the patients who were misdiagnosed sought mental health treatment before learning they really were having PSVT episodes.

Archives of Internal Medicine, March 10, 1997.

Millions are spent each year on unnecessary pap smears

For years, the medical establishment has been criticized for performing millions of unnecessary hysterectomies yet it is still the most frequent surgical procedure inflicted on females.

By the time a woman reaches age 50, her chances of having had a hysterectomy are one in three — 4.6 hysterectomies are performed every minute during business hours in the U.S. Often, the woman is not even informed about safe and effective alternatives.

A study published in *The New England Journal of Medicine* showed that even after the hysterectomy, most women are told they should continue to get annual pap smears to detect vaginal cancer. However, the disease is almost non-existent in women who have had hysterectomies since the cervix is removed.

Pap smears are pumping millions of dollars into the pockets of medical doctors who are either ignorant about this type of cancer or are motivated by monetary considerations rather than the welfare of their patients. More than 13% of all pap smears performed in the U.S. are in women who have had hysterectomies.

"Eliminating pap smears for women who have had a hysterectomy as a result of a benign disorder would result in big savings for our healthcare system," explained researcher Dr. Katherine Pearce.

"For the future of women's health, hopefully the results of this study will help redirect the dollars that are being spent on this unnecessary task and put them toward something to truly benefit women," she said.

This is not the first time doctors have been apprised that pap smears are not needed for women who have had a hysterectomy. After reviewing more than 70 studies, researchers from the University of Michigan reached a similar conclusion.

SOURCES: "Cytopathological findings on vaginal Papanicolaou smears after hysterectomy for benign gynecologic disease," by Katherine F. Pearce, Hope K. Haefner, Syeda F. Sarwar, and Thomas E. Nolan. *The New England Journal of Medicine (NEJM)*, November 21, 1996.

"PAP smears for some women could become thing of the past," *Cancer Weekly Plus*, December 9, 1996.

"Pap smears after hysterectomy," *Harvard Health Letter*, August 1996.

In-home drug delivery system blasted by women's health group

The National Women's Health Network (NWHN) asked the Food & Drug Administration (FDA) to take the Matria Healthcare drug pump off the market after two women lost their lives using it.

According to the women's health advocacy group, the pump administers an asthma drug called terbutaline that was being prescribed for pregnant women to avoid premature labor — even though the drug had NOT been approved for that purpose. In addition, the drug's label warned that it can cause "serious adverse reactions" and "maternal deaths" and was specific in noting that it "should not be used for the management of premature labor."

At least two women died after using the pump and eight others suffered heart or lung problems because of the terbutaline. One baby was born with heart damage, which doctors linked to the drug use.

"The worst thing that would happen if this technology weren't used was that the babies might die," stated Cynthia Pearson, executive director of the NWHN. "That would be terrible ... to lose both the baby and the mother is just a million times worse, and that's what this is putting women at risk of."

The company which rents out the drug pump — Matria Healthcare — refused to assume responsibility for the deaths declaring, "We're caught in the middle — we don't own the drug."

But the NWHN, although not actually faulting the pump itself, stated the in-home delivery system of a mis-prescribed drug puts pregnant women at greater risk and, therefore, should be removed from the market.

SOURCE: "Health advocates attack premature labor pump," Associated Press, July 1, 1996.

M.D.s underestimate steroid osteoporosis risk

One of the most dangerous side effects of corticosteroid use is osteoporosis. Yet, a survey presented at a national meeting of the American College of Rheumatology (ACR) showed that many physicians don't realize it! The survey of physicians was conducted by researchers at the Medical College of Virginia/Virginia Commonwealth University.

According to the ACR, corticosteroids (different from the steroids sometimes used by athletes to enhance performance) are prescribed by a wide range of physicians of varying specialties and training.

The drugs are prescribed for patients with serious autoimmune diseases like lupus or rheumatoid arthritis, "but the side effects can sometimes be worse than the disease itself," the ACR stated. Other diseases for which steroids are commonly used include asthma, chronic lung disease and inflammatory bowel disease.

Although males and pre-menopausal women are generally considered to be at low risk for developing osteoporosis, long-term steroid use can greatly increase their risk over time. Nevertheless, while many of the doctors surveyed indicated that they were aware of the possibility that steroids could cause osteoporosis, they didn't feel the risk was particularly great.

"If steroid-induced bone loss is to be prevented, better education about the risks and treatments for patients on steroids is needed," said Lenore M. Buckley, M.D., MPH, lead author of the survey.

Source:"Physicians lack understanding of osteoporosis risk with steroids," American College of Rheumatology, October 13, 1996.

Chapter 15

The cruelest cut of all

Cutting a body open and physically removing parts of it is the ultimate insult to the human system. Once, it was considered only as a last resort, a desperate measure to be taken when all else failed. Today, people routinely go under the knife for everything from cancer to cosmetic reasons. They willingly permit themselves to be drugged into unconsciousness and subjected to procedures which are often of dubious effectiveness — and frequently pose grave health risks in and of themselves.

Although it embraces new technology, the medical profession has a tendency to reject new ideas. Surgeons are willing to learn new ways of performing operations, although few seem eager to examine possible alternatives to surgery. Much of this can of course be explained by the fact that research into surgery is normally performed by surgeons. Their training and experience does not lend itself to looking into other options. Cardiac surgeons, for instance, would be unlikely to work at a project that would prove that most heart operations are unnecessary or dangerous. That conclusion would not only put their livelihood at risk, but also invalidate their entire vocation.

The only people in the operating room who have a clear reason for wanting the truth are the patients on the tables. But if we wait until that moment to learn the truth, it might be too late.

More than half of all surgeries may be unnecessary

Any lawyer will tell you that the hardest thing to find in a medical malpractice case is an M.D. willing to testify against a colleague. It's little wonder, then, that few studies have been done by the medical establishment which might reveal the number of unnecessary surgeries performed each year in this country.

In his book, "Health Shock," journalist Martin Weitz reported that a 1974 Senate investigation into unnecessary surgery found that "American doctors performed 2.4 million unnecessary operations, causing 11,900 deaths and costing $3.9 billion."

In 1982, Robert G. Schneider, M.D., calculated that between 15 and 25% of all surgeries were unnecessary — with that figure rising to 50-60% with some types of operations. In the case of tonsillectomies and hysterectomies, the percentage was as high as 40-80%.

But a search of the massive Health Database Plus — with 274,449 articles published in thousands of health magazines and journals — yielded only 55 (far fewer than 1% of the total) under the key words "unnecessary surgeries." And, most of those were in non-medical consumer health care publications.

Despite what appears to be an attempt by the medical profession to keep that kind of information from the public, a few reports have surfaced which show clearly that the problem with unnecessary surgeries is not a thing of the past.

In a 1995 report issued by Milliman & Robertson, Inc., titled "Analysis of Medically Unnecessary Inpatient Services," researchers David V. Axene, FSA and Richard Doyle, M.D., concluded that "the level of medically unnecessary use may actually be closer to 60%" (than their previously projected 53%). This included a variety of surgical procedures as well as associated services.

That same year, the federal government's Agency for Health Care Policy Research (AHCPR) concluded that most back surgery was unnecessary. Back surgeons immediately began a campaign to abolish the agency.

Other reports confirm this frightening statistic.

A report in *Medical Update* noted that, "Every year, American surgeons perform about a quarter of a million appendectomies for suspected appendicitis — about 20 percent of which turn out to be unnecessary."

The situation with hysterectomies is even worse. Up to one third of all surgeries may be unnecessary, according to a 1990 research report by Blue Cross/Blue Shield of Illinois. A 1993 RAND Institute Study, published in the *Journal of the American Medical Association (JAMA)*, concluded that 10-27% of hysterectomies were judged to be "inappropriate" and another 24% were of uncertain benefit.

The enormity of this problem becomes apparent when it is noted that over half a million women are subjected each year to a hysterectomy for benign female reproductive disorders that are not life-threatening.

Obviously, despite the shortage of reports from the medical profession itself, the problem of unnecessary surgeries is still a serious one. Yet, ironically, unnecessary surgery normally is not considered medical malpractice.

According to "Medicine on Trial," a People's Medical Society book: "When greed controls the impulse to operate when an operation is not called for, as is often the case in unnecessary surgery, such an operation is certainly a grossly unethical and immoral act, but not a medical mistake per se."

The ultimate solution is prevention. But when, as a last resort, surgery must be considered, patients need to have full and honest information about the risks and benefits involved in the procedure.

The People's Medical Society has warned: "as long as the medical profession covers up for its faulty own ... surgery will be a crap shoot for the person who needs it or thinks he needs it."

SOURCES: "Analysis of Medically Unnecessary Inpatient Services," by David Axene, FSA and Richard Doyle, M.D. Milliman & Robertson, Inc., 1995.

"Health Shock," by Martin Weitz. Prentice-Hall. 1982.

"When to Say No to Surgery," by Robert G. Schneider, M.D. Prentice-Hall, 1982.

"Entrenched medical practices: time to take action," *HealthFacts*, August 1990.

"50,000 unnecessary appendectomies a year — and how to prevent them," by Edwin W. Brown, *Medical Update*, Feb. 1997.

"Federal agency under fire: finds most back surgery unnecessary," *HealthFacts*, Oct. 1995.

"Unnecessary hysterectomy: the controversy that will not die." *HealthFacts*, July 1993.

"Hysterectomy: overused or appropriately performed?," by Barbara Apgar, *American Family Physician*, Feb. 15, 1997.

"Medicine On Trial," by Charles B. Inlander, et. al., People's Medical Society, 1988.

M.D.s lacking angioplasty experience costing patients their lives

More than half of all U.S. physicians who performed coronary angioplasty in 1992 did not have the minimum amount of experience in the procedure, as established in 1988 by the American Heart Association (AHA) and the American College of Cardiology (ACC), according to Durham, N.C. researchers who studied medical records of 97,491 Medicare patients.

Coronary angioplasty is a non-surgical but invasive procedure in which a catheter tipped with a tiny un-inflated balloon is passed through the body's circulatory system to a severely narrowed section of a blood vessel.

When the balloon is inflated it crushes the deposits of cholesterol and other fatty material against the vessel wall, opening the channel for blood to flow.

In addition, Duke University Medical Center investigators, headed by James G. Jollis, M.D., revealed another alarming fact at the American Heart Association's 69th Scientific Sessions. Patients of physicians who performed fewer of the balloon catheter procedures were more likely to wind up under the surgeon's knife or become a cardiac fatality.

"Our findings show that the AHA and ACC guidelines should be followed," said Jollis, "and that physicians who perform fewer than the recommended number of angioplasties per year have a higher percentage of patients who go on to have bypass surgery or die."

The situation presents a "Catch 22" for patients, however. Since Jollis advised patients who are considering undergoing the procedure to judge their physician by how many angioplasties he or she performs, the findings may create a "more is better" attitude among doctors wishing to perform the costly procedure.

SOURCE:"Most physicians performing angioplasty fail to meet minimum standards — and their patients fare worse," press release from Dr. James G.

Jollis. Nov. 13, 1996. Original paper presented at American Heart Association's 69th Scientific Sessions.

Bypass patients risk neurological damage

The coronary bypass procedure, which is supposed to save lives, may actually cause neurological damage in some patients. That was the news presented during a meeting of the American Neurological Association in San Diego, California.

It is well known that bypass patients often experience memory problems such as difficulty recognizing familiar faces, reading, or remembering recent events. But most medical researchers thought these were temporary reactions which faded in a few months.

A research project by Dr. Ola A. Selnes, associate professor of neurology at the Johns Hopkins University School of Medicine, revealed that these complaints of feeling "cobwebs in the head" were still evident in many bypass patients in the Johns Hopkins study five years after the procedure.

In the small, long-term study, 99 patients were given a battery of psychological and neurological tests prior to their bypass surgery, and then one month, one year, and five years after the procedure.

Five years after the surgery, 23% of the patients showed an abnormal decline in their cognitive ability, such as remembering visual images, compared to tests taken earlier; 18% showed an abnormal decline in their ability to deal with spatial relations; 16% had abnormal difficulty remembering words; 12% had language difficulties; and 9% showed evidence of attention deficit.

Dr. Selnes said that such neurological problems exceed those that could be attributed to aging, depression or even Alzheimer's disease. Unless a problem occurs, normal elderly people have stable cognitive abilities.

The research will undoubtedly rekindle the debate about the controversial procedure, which critics say is overused. According to the American Heart Association, in 1994 doctors in the U.S. performed about 501,000 bypass procedures on about 318,000 patients.

SOURCES: La Voie, Angela: "Bypass Surgery May Cause Neurological Problems," *Medical Tribune News Service,* The New York Times, October 1, 1997.

"Bypass Patients Suffer Cognitive Impairments," *Reuters Health Information Services, Inc.,* October 3, 1997.

Some cardiac procedures don't help

U.S. physicians have built a world-wide reputation of performing far more surgeries than their colleagues in other countries. Now, there is more evidence that many of those operations aren't helping patients.

Researchers from Harvard Medical School and the Institute for Clinical Evaluative Sciences in Canada found that U.S. physicians performed many more invasive cardiac procedures to treat elderly heart-attack patients than did Canadian physicians — but their patients were just as likely to die within one year as those in Canada.

The one-year mortality rates were 34.3% for Americans and 34.4% for Canadians. Even the short-term benefits of these procedures are not particularly significant: when death rates were measured for 30 days — 21.4% of Americans died and 22.3% of Canadians — suggesting only a small, short-term edge for American cardiac care.

The researchers concluded that despite this small, short-term advantage, the data overall seem to favor the more conservative Canadian practices.

The research team looked at patients age 65 and older in the U.S. and Canada who had suffered a new myocardial infarction in 1991. Myocardial infarction, or heart attack, is a leading cause of death and disease in both the U.S. and Canada. The team compared the use of three cardiac procedures within 30 days of the attack and patient mortality rates in the two countries.

The procedures were coronary angiography, a diagnostic technique using a contrast medium to produce X-ray images of the coronary arteries; percutaneous transluminal coronary angioplasty, insertion of a balloon catheter through the skin and into the channel of a coronary artery to dilate a narrowed section of the artery by inflating the balloon; and coronary-artery bypass graft surgery, a procedure to graft a section of vein between the aorta and a blocked coronary artery to reroute blood flow around the obstruction.

The subjects included 224,258 elderly Medicare recipients in the U.S. and 9,444 elderly patients in Ontario. The study found that the Americans were much more likely to undergo the invasive procedures: For coronary angiography, the figures were 34.9% of the American patients vs. 6.7% of the Canadians; for percutaneous transluminal coronary angioplasty, 11.7% vs. 1.5% and for coronary-artery bypass graft surgery, 10.6% vs. 1.4%

The differences in use of the procedures decreased only a small amount during 180 days of follow-up.

"The results of our study are likely to stimulate debate about the costs and effectiveness of the more aggressive U.S. approach," wrote lead author Jack V. Tu, Barbara McNeil, and colleagues. Tu was in the Department of Health Care Policy at Harvard Medical School (HMS) at the time of the study and McNeil is chair of the department and the Ridley Watts Professor of Health Care Policy.

In an accompanying editorial, Harlan M. Krumholz of Yale University School of Medicine pointed out that no other country in the world matches the rate of cardiac procedures performed in the U.S., rates that have grown dramatically since 1980.

"The relatively high rate of use of procedures may have been fostered by a health care delivery system that, until recently, almost uniformly favored their use," he wrote.

SOURCE: *The New England Journal of Medicine,* May 22, 1997.

Chapter 16

Researching the Truth

M any of the reports in this book are based on studies published in scientific and medical research journals. In the past, these publications could be relied upon to present research papers even if the outcomes were critical of certain procedures or drugs.

However, in more recent years, the tentacles of big business have reached into and infected even the more reputable research centers and publications. Research projects are routinely funded or conducted by drug companies, and medical organizations and their journals rely heavily on revenues from pharmaceutical advertising.

We must, therefore, be skeptical whenever we read of a new medical "miracle." That miracle is, to drug companies and the medical industry, just another product to be marketed for the highest profit possible.

Medical research often suppressed by drug makers

Medical researchers have long protected their image as dedicated and caring scientists who only want to help humanity.

That image was badly tarnished after the release of a 1997 study, published in *Journal of the American Medical Association (JAMA),* which disclosed that nearly one out of every five researchers actually withhold their research in order to maximize their profits. In some cases, the research was suppressed by drug manufacturing companies which were unhappy with the results of the research they funded.

David Blumenthal, M.D., MPP, from Massachusetts General Hospital Partners Health Care System and Boston's Harvard Medical School and colleagues surveyed 3,394 life-science faculty from the 50 universities which received the most funding from the National Institutes of Health in 1993. Sixty-four percent (2,167) of those 3,394 responded.

Of those, 410 (19.8%) admitted that publication of their research results had been delayed by more than six months in the last three years at least once. Although they are supposed to be motivated by a desire to improve the health of all people, they had a variety of unethical reasons for keeping their findings a secret. The reasons given for delaying the release of the information included:

➤ 46% to allow time to apply for patents;

➤ 33% to protect the proprietary value of research results by means other than patent applications;

➤ 31% to protect their scientific lead;

➤ 28% to slow dissemination of undesired results;

➤ 26% to allow time to negotiate license agreements; and

➤ 17% to resolve disputes over intellectual property.

Among faculty who were involved in commercialization of their research, 31% reported publication delays **longer than six months.**

Another myth that was shattered by the report was that all scientists are willing to work together for the common good. The survey showed that self-ishness was a factor in the scientific community — 181 respondents admitting that they had refused to share research results or materials with other univer-sity scientists in the last three years.

Of those refusing to share, 46% did so to protect their scientific lead, 27% because of the limited supply or high costs of the materials requested; 18% because of a previous informal agreement with a company; 6% to protect the financial interest of the university; 4% because of a formal agreement with a company; and 2% to protect their own financial interests in the results of their research.

The researchers who conducted the survey noted: "The power of the ideal of openness is reflected in the following quotation from Albert Einstein, inscribed on his statue in front of the headquarters of the National Academy of Sciences: 'The right to search for truth implies also a duty: one must not con-ceal any part of what one has recognized to be true.'

"Nevertheless," the researchers continued, "strong pressures, both personal and external to researchers, may result in their breaching of the ideal of open-ness. Personal pressures include competition between researchers for priority and recognition. External pressures include the requirements of the promotion process, competition for funding, and processes and procedures related to the commercialization of university research."

The same issue of *JAMA* contained a research article on thyroid medications which had been suppressed since its completion in 1990.

In a separate editorial, Drummond Rennie, M.D., deputy editor (West) of *JAMA,* explained that the original research into various thyroid medications was contracted by Flint Laboratories, which manufactured a thyroid drug called Synthroid. They hired a pharmacology researcher, Betty J. Dong, Pharm.D., from University of California at San Francisco, who shared their belief that the study would prove Synthroid was superior to its competitors. Although Flint was taken over by another drug maker, Boots Pharmaceutical, Inc., the research continued.

When Dong's research actually showed that it was no better than any of the oth-ers, Boots tried to discredit her and her study. The research paper was eventually submitted to *JAMA* over Boots' objections, but was withdrawn by Dong before it went to press. She cited 'impending legal action by Boots Pharmaceuticals, Inc. against UCSF and the investigators,' as the reason for her action.

The FDA notified Synthroid's manufacturer (now a company called Knoll Pharmaceutical) that its claim that its drug was superior to other preparations was misleading. On November 7, 1996, the FDA concluded that Knoll had violated federal law. A few weeks later, Knoll agreed not to block publication of the manuscript, although they still insist that the researcher's conclusions are not supported by the data.

SOURCES: "Thyroid Storm," by Drummond Rennie. *The Journal of the American Medical Association*, April 16, 1997.

"Withholding research results in academic life science: evidence from a national survey of faculty," by David Blumenthal, et al. *The Journal of the American Medical Association*, April 16, 1997.

Medical journal authors found to be drug company consultants

Numerous health professionals have been warning the public about the possible dangers of the newly approved appetite suppressant dexfenfluramine, manufactured by Interneuron Pharmaceutical Inc. and sold under the trade name of "Redux." Studies have linked the drug to the potentially deadly condition pulmonary hypertension, as well as sleep disorders and depression.

That's why many were surprised to read a favorable article about the drug in the *New England Journal of Medicine (NEJM)*.

It wasn't until later that the authors of the article were discovered to be paid consultants to the firms making and marketing the drug. *NEJM's* editor, Marcia Angell, said that the authors had not properly revealed their links with the pharmaceutical company when they submitted the article.

The article claimed the benefits of fenfluramine and its derivatives outweigh the side effects - - even though almost one-third of the 95 people with pulmonary hypertension included in the study had been taking fenfluramine. This translated to a risk 23 times greater than in people who don't use the diet pill, they admitted.

Still, the authors argued the drug could save an estimated 280 lives for every million persons treated. They also claimed that the drug would cause an estimated 14 deaths for every one million persons treated. This was later found to be inaccurate and the figures were increased to 46 out of every million.

Previously, authors JoAnn E. Manson, a Harvard Medical School associate professor, and Gerald A. Faich, adjunct professor at the University of Pennsylvania Medical School, had been paid to testify before the FDA in order to win approval for the drug.

Stock for Interneuron rose by nearly 13% as soon as the favorable article was published. The stock of American Home Products Corp., which markets the drug, rose by more than two percent.

Angell said the journal's editors were led to believe the authors worked for the government and the situation would be "looked into." She also suggested that the journal might "make readers aware of the situation," in a future issue.

SOURCES: "Pharmacotherapy for obesity — do the benefits outweigh the risks?" by JoAnn E. Manson and Gerald A. Faich, *The New England Journal of Medicine,* August 29, 1996 v335 n9 p659(2).

"Medical journal says it was misled by writers," Associated Press. August 28, 1996.

Study on cholesterol drug funded by drug maker

A 1996 study concluded that hundreds of thousands of deaths and repeat heart attacks could be avoided if patients *with normal cholesterol levels* were given prescriptions for the drug "Pravachol."

Yet, many health care observers remained skeptical about the research since the $42 million project had been **paid for** by Bristol-Myers Squibb, the maker of Pravachol.

"The message is that if you have a **high** risk of heart attack, your *exact* level of cholesterol is not too important. It's probably too high for you," said one of the researchers, Dr. Terje R. Pederson of Aker Hospital in Oslo, Norway. (emphases added)

Treatment with Pravachol costs an estimated $750-900 annually and researchers admitted it would take at least two years of treatment to experience any benefit.

A quick calculation arrives at another possible motive for the drug maker's endorsement of the drug. Treatment of just 200,000 people would mean an estimated annual revenue of about $165 million.

SOURCES: "Drugs aid 'ordinary cholesterol'," Associated Press, March 27, 1996.

Medical journal ethics still questioned

In 1996, the *New England Journal of Medicine (NEJM)* came under fire after it published an article putting the newly approved appetite suppressant *dexfenfluramine* (known as "Redux") in a positive light despite numerous studies showing its risks outweighed any benefits. Later, it was revealed that the pro-Redux article was written by two paid consultants to the firms which manufactured and sold the drug.

The incident, which made many people question the integrity or at least the conscientiousness of the journal, is still being discussed in the medical community.

At the time, Britain's top medical journal, *The Lancet,* refused to condemn its American cousin, stating that it was "sympathetic," because, like the *NEJM* it has to rely on "the conscience and judgement of the author to draw our attention to such a personal conflict."

But in an issue of *The Lancet, NEJM's* ethics were again questioned when a British cardiologist wrote about a similar situation that had happened several years ago.

According to Dr. Peter Wilmshurst, an article about a drug called *amrinone* had been published, with "all five authors listed as employees of hospitals associated with Harvard Medical School when two were employees of Sterling [the company which made amrinone], and two others, including a member of the *NEJM* editorial board, were paid consultants to the company."

Lancet editors noted that this "allegation of undeclared conflict of interest between individuals connected with the *NEJM* and Sterling was a serious one implying that the *NEJM* may not have judged the suitability of the article for publication entirely on grounds of scientific merit."

In his letter to the editor, Dr. Wilmshurst said: "I asked the Massachusetts Medical Society [owners of the journal] to investigate specific complaints. They refused. I asked the *NEJM* to publish my letter on the subject together with a response. It refused."

Which, at the very least, leaves many people questioning how many of the pro-drug articles published in the *NEJM* are actually little more than advertisements.

SOURCES: "Medical journal says it was misled by writers," Associated Press. August 28, 1996.

New England Journal of Medicine, August 29, 1996, v335 n9, p659(2).

The Lancet, February 15, 1997.

Chapter 17

The high blood pressure scam

High blood pressure — also called hypertension — is a true health risk. But it didn't really become a "silent killer" until the medical profession began treating it with dangerous drugs and questionable therapies.

Scientific and medical research have clearly shown that most cases of hypertension can be effectively treated and eliminated through proper life style changes — diet, exercise, chiropractic and relaxation techniques. Yet, few medical doctors try any of those approaches with their patients. Instead, they prescribe drugs which can make the situation worse, cause other equally or more serious health problems and subject the person to dangerous and even life-threatening side effects.

Blood pressure drugs may do more harm than good

The potential benefits of taking medication to lower high blood pressure (antihypertensives) may not outweigh their negative effects on quality of life for some patients, reports a study funded in part by the U.S. Department of Health and Human Services' Agency for Health Care Policy and Research.

Side effects of these medications include fatigue, weakness, headache, joint and stomach aches, nausea, impotence, and urinary tract problems. Often, the reduction in blood pressure was not significant for some patients, despite the numerous side effects caused by the drugs.

Researchers from the University of Wisconsin at Madison interviewed 1,430 randomly selected adults 45-89 years old. They obtained medical histories and measured the subjects' health status using a variety of measures and self reports.

Of those interviewed, 519 reported being affected by hypertension for more than three years. Persons with hypertension scored lower on the "overall health" test than those whose blood pressure was normal.

But, of the people with high blood pressure, those taking increasing numbers of antihypertensive drugs scored the lowest of all.

SOURCE: "Health status and hypertension: A population-based study," by William F. Lawrence, M.D., M.S.; Dennis G. Fryback, Ph.D.; Patricia A. Martin, M.A, and others, *Journal of Clinical Epidemiology,* November 1996.

Channel blockers pose threats to HBP patients

Calcium channel blockers make up one of the most widely prescribed class of drugs for high blood pressure in the world. Yet, research has shown that these drugs can increase the risk of heart attacks and gastrointestinal bleeding. And two medical studies have suggested that the drugs may be even more dangerous than doctors had realized.

A report in the *Journal of the American Medical Association (JAMA)*, concluded that people being treated for high blood pressure with the short-acting calcium channel blocker "isradipine" may be at greater risk for major vascular events such as heart attack or stroke compared to treatment with a diuretic.

Michele Mercuri, M.D., Ph.D., from the Division of Vascular Ultrasound Research, The Bowman Gray School of Medicine, Winston-Salem, N.C., and colleagues made the finding while comparing the two therapies in the treatment of carotid artery disease in hypertensive patients.

The study included 883 patients from nine medical centers. The patients received twice daily doses of isradipine or the diuretic hydrochlorothiazide. Researchers conducted the study in order to measure the progression of the thickening of any of the four principal (carotid) arteries of the neck and head in patients taking the two drugs.

The researchers found a higher incidence of major vascular events (myocardial infarction, stroke, congestive heart failure, angina, and sudden death) in isradipine patients when compared with patients taking hydrochlorothiazide.

They also found a significant increase in non-major vascular problems.

In an accompanying editorial, Aram V. Chobanian, M.D., Boston University School of Medicine, noted: "Short-acting dihydropyridine derivatives (i.e., isradipine) clearly should be avoided in the vast majority of patients with cardiovascular diseases, including hypertension."

In another study — reported in the British Medical Journal *The Lancet* — researchers found that use of the calcium channel blockers may be linked to higher rates of cancer.

The study involved more than 5,000 people aged 71 and older. Researchers concluded that the risk of developing cancer was 72% higher among those who used the short-acting forms of calcium channel blockers.

The drugs — manufactured by several pharmaceutical companies including Bayer and Pfizer, Inc. — had already been criticized because they were not subjected to scientifically rigorous trials before winning approval. Those studies are in process but not expected to be completed for some time.

Not all doctors — or drug manufacturers — are willing to believe the medication is as dangerous as these research studies have seemed to indicate. Some medical journals have even called for a "moratorium" on publishing any more negative reports — a move which was criticized by the editor of *The Lancet*.

In order to counter the negative publicity, an Israeli researcher issued a news release to coincide with *The Lancet* report. In it, he claimed that his own unpublished research showed no increased risk of cancer from taking the drug. Hardly a comforting development when, according to an article in *The New York Times*, "Bayer, the maker of one calcium channel blocker, helped write and distribute the news release about his findings."

Releasing information on a research project before the findings are reviewed and published is considered highly irregular in scientific circles.

The dispute became so intense the FBI began looking into death threats sent to doctors involved, *The Lancet* editorial noted.

SOURCES: Journal of the American Medical Association (JAMA), September 10, 1996.

"Short-acting calcium channel blocker may trigger cardiovascular problems," AMA media advisory, September 10, 1996.

"Calcium-channel blockade and incidence of cancer in aged populations," *The Lancet*, August 24, 1996.

"Blood Pressure Drug Linked to Cancer in Elderly," by Lawrence K. Altman, *The New York Times*, August 23, 1996.

Common blood pressure drug linked to breast cancer risk

Despite mounting proof that the best way to reduce blood pressure is diet and lifestyle, many medical doctors continue to prescribe drugs, including calcium channel blockers.

However, a study published in the October 15, 1997 issue of *Cancer* shows a possible link between those drugs and a greatly increased risk of breast cancer in postmenopausal women. The risk is even greater in those women who also take estrogen replacement therapy.

According to the research project results, taking calcium channel blockers made the women's risk of developing breast cancer twice as high as that of older women taking no blood pressure drugs.

Calcium channel blockers are prescribed to treat high blood pressure and heart disease. They include drugs such as Cardizem, Adalat, Procardia, diltiazem, verapamil, and nifedipine.

Researcher Dr. Annette Fitzpatrick of the University of Washington in Seattle directed the investigation, which included 3,198 women, aged 65-100.

During the course of the study, women developed 75 cases of breast cancer. Researchers found that women taking calcium channel blockers had twice the risk of developing breast cancer than those taking other types of blood pressure drugs or no blood pressure drugs at all. Women taking estrogen replacement therapy as well as calcium channel blockers seemed to have the highest risk.

SOURCES: "Use of Calcium Channel Blockers and Breast Carcinoma Risk in Postmenopausal Women," *Cancer*, October 15, 1997.

"Calcium Channel Blockers and Breast Cancer Risk," NIH Statement, October 14, 1997.

M.D.s continued prescribing antihypertensive agent despite FDA disapproval

Despite the fact that the Food & Drug Administration (FDA) had not approved *nifedipine* capsules for treatment of hypertensive conditions, medical doctors continued to administer them to patients.

Physicians appeared to ignore information showing that use may result in serious adverse effects ranging from severe low blood pressure, stroke, and heart attack to death.

That was the conclusion of medical researchers who conducted a literature review on the practice of giving nifedipine in hypertensive emergencies and pseudo-emergencies.

A "hypertensive emergency" is defined as severely elevated blood pressure accompanied by target organ disease such as stroke, acute renal failure or heart attack. A "hypertensive pseudo-emergency" is defined as severe blood pressure elevation, presumably chronic, without evidence of target organ disease.

Nifedipine, in the form of short-acting capsules given orally or under the tongue, continues to be a common treatment for hypertensive emergencies and pseudoemergencies according to a report in *The Journal of the American Medial Association (JAMA)*.

In 1985, members of the FDA's Cardiorenal Advisory Committee unanimously rejected nifedipine capsules for this use because of the lack of outcome data.

The researchers noted: "Just because the practice of giving oral nifedipine capsules in hypertensive emergencies and pseudoemergencies is widespread and popular does not mean that it is safe and effective. To the contrary, serious — even fatal — adverse effects have been reported when the drug has been administered acutely for treatment of severe hypertension."

The authors explained that the use of nifedipine for the "cosmetic" purpose of correcting blood pressure does not help the patient and may turn a pseudo-emergency into a real emergency when blood pressure is dramatically lowered.

SOURCES:The Journal of the American Medical Association (JAMA), October 23/30, 1996.

Media advisory, American Medical Association, October 18, 1996.

Hypertension drugs may increase risk of cancer, heart attack, death

In the August 1996 issue of *Health Watch,* we reported on a study which showed that for most people, drug therapy to lower high blood pressure doesn't work. In essence, Americans are throwing billions of dollars down the drain every year on useless medications.

We since learned of studies which are even more alarming, because they show that some of those medicines may violate the Hippocratic Oath to "do no harm." In fact, two research projects produced evidence that calcium channel blockers — frequently prescribed to patients with high blood pressure — might *increase* the person's risk of getting cancer, as well as having a heart attack.

A compilation of 16 prior studies had indicated that several of the calcium channel blockers actually tripled a patient's risk of death, compared to a placebo.

The first research results were presented at the March 10, 1995 meeting of the Epidemiology and Prevention Council of the American Heart Association.

The conclusion drawn from a study of 291 patients was that calcium-channel blockers used as antihypertensive agents appeared to increase the risk of myocardial infarction even in otherwise healthy hypertensive patients.

A previous study had shown the drugs could increase the risk for those who had already suffered a heart attack, but this project uncovered the increased risk for all people.

A report published in the *American Journal of Hypertension* revealed that those same calcium-channel blockers might also increase the risk of cancer. The incidence of cancer for research subjects who were taking the drug was twice as high as for those not on the channel-blockers. The subjects were all age 71 or older.

An estimated six million American take calcium channel blockers, spending about $3.5 billion on the drugs each year. A spokesperson for Pfizer, Inc., which sells the lucrative calcium-channel blocker Procardia, strongly criticized the report.

One criticism leveled at the early study was that it involved only an older version of the drug, which accounted for about 10% of the total drug usage. The principal researcher admitted that the study involved only the older type, but expressed doubt that the new "one- a-day" drugs would prove any safer.

"If you have a toxic substance and put it into a long-release, it's still a toxic substance," noted Dr. Curt Furberg, one of the authors of the research study.

Although this was the third major research study to provide evidence that this class of drugs may greatly increase people's risk for both heart attacks and cancer, the medical and pharmaceutical industries urged patients not to discontinue taking the medicine. They are also being encouraged to consult their doctors (presumably the same ones who prescribed the drug in the first place) about the potential risks, and are being warned that sudden withdrawal of these drugs can be fatal.

The FDA has taken no steps to remove the drugs from the market.

SOURCES: "Calcium-channel Blockers Under Fire", *Medical Sciences Bulletin.* April 1995.

Research paper, Curt Furberg, M.D. and Bruce Psaty, M.D. Epidemiology and Prevention Council of the American Heart Association meeting, March 10, 1995. San Antonio, Texas.

Research paper by Dr. Richard Havlik, et. al. *American Journal of Hypertension,* July 1996.

"Medication may increase cancer risk, study suggests." Associated Press. June 26, 1996.

"Study links some hypertension drugs to cancer risk." Bloomberg News Service. June 26, 1996.

Medical approach to treating hypertension has failed

Millions of dollars have been pumped into creating new drugs to treat high blood pressure, the most common risk factor for the leading cause of death in the U.S. — heart disease. Thousands of prescriptions are written each month for drugs which are supposed to lower blood pressure, but it's clear now that this medical approach has failed.

According to an article in *The Journal of the American Medical Association (JAMA)*, for most people, the drug therapy doesn't work.

William B. Kannel, M.D., Boston University School of Medicine, studied a group of subjects over a four-decade period for signs of heart disease in relation to their blood pressure and other suspected risk factors.

Dr. Kannel cited information that approximately 50 million Americans, or one in four adults, have high blood pressure. Each year, about two million people are diagnosed as hypertensive. One-third are unaware they are hypertensive. Only 21% of those under treatment have their blood pressure under good control.

Hypertension has been found to be a strong predisposing factor in heart attacks, strokes and artery disease. Hypertension usually occurs along with other risk factors such as smoking, diabetes and obesity.

Dr. Kannel found no evidence of a decline in hypertension, defined as blood pressure greater than 140/90 millimeters of mercury (mm Hg). In fact, he found an increase in blood pressure of about 20/10 mm Hg among participants age 30-to-65.

He noted, "The absence of a decline in prevalence of hypertension indicates an urgent need for primary prevention by weight control, exercise, and reduced salt and alcohol intake."

However, his suggestions for a prevention program unintentionally proved the medical profession doesn't yet understand the causes of hypertension. To highlight the point, another article in the same issue concluded that reducing salt in the diet has only a "non-significant" effect on blood pressure.

SOURCES"The progression from hypertension to congestive heart failure.," *The Journal of the American Medical Association (JAMA)*, May 22, 1996 v275 n20 p1557(6).

"Blood pressure as a cardiovascular risk factor: prevention and treatment," *JAMA, The Journal of the American Medical Association*, May 22, 1996 v275 n20 p1571(6).

Chapter 18

Capsules of gold

I f medication was given away for free — or if there were price limits on drugs — the number of prescriptions written in this country would drop tremendously. But in our free market economy, pushing pills (even the legal, prescription and over-the-counter type) is one of the most profitable businesses around.

This has led to having dangerous and sometimes potentially deadly drugs marketed like breakfast cereal or athletic shoes: celebrity endorsements, glitzy television ads, coupons, special promotions, and full page magazine spreads.

The fact that these promotions can be misleading doesn't seem to deter drug company executives, who judge their success solely on their bottom line — without regard to the health and welfare of the people who are lured into taking their products.

Drug company broadcasts misleading television ads

Less than two weeks after the Food & Drug Administration (FDA) relaxed the rules for drug ads on television, drug maker Schering-Plough crossed the line and broadcast two ads which failed to give a balanced look at both the possible benefits and potential dangers for the product.

The drug in question is *Claritin,* a popular antihistamine which is available by prescription only and which has been heavily marketed in print ads.

The FDA reprimanded the company and cited it for violation of two regulations, saying that "both advertisements are misleading because the risk information disclosed as part of the required 'major statement' is not presented in a manner comparable to that used to present the information relating to efficacy." The agency asked Schering to "immediately discontinue the use of the advertisement[s]."

The first part of the 30-second ads contained the "pro" information — in clear, easy-to- understand language. The information about negative side effects was read so rapidly that most people wouldn't be able to understand it. In addition, an unrelated message was displayed on the screen, making it even more difficult to get a true picture of the drug's dangers.

In one ad, consumers were referred to a *Newsweek* magazine advertisement for details on the drug, while in the other, they were given the company's internet address as a source of more information.

According to a statement issued by Larry Sasich, Pharm.D., M.P.H. and Sidney M. Wolfe, M.D., of Public Citizen's Health Research Group, the relaxed FDA regulations serve only to increase drug sales — not educate the public.

"The drug industry loves the new guidelines," they said. "Alan F. Holmer, president of the Pharmaceutical Research and Manufacturers of America, a drug industry trade group, is quoted as saying the FDA was 'striking a blow for patients.' The only blow that has been struck has been against consumers who still have no easily available, objective source of comprehensive adverse reaction information about prescription drugs and, instead, are going to be barraged with an increasing crescendo of false and misleading information on TV and in DTC print ads."

SOURCES: Food and Drug Administration letter to Schering-Plough Corp., August 19, 1997.

"Schering broadcasts misleading loratadine (Claritin) direct-to-consumer TV ads," Public Citizen's Health Research Group, August 20, 1997.

Drug makers exploit patient emotions

A study in the *British Medical Journal* confirmed what consumers have known for years: drug companies play on the emotions of patients rather than help them make logical decisions about what medications to take.

"Advertisers are increasingly using symbols to circumvent logical argument when trying to persuade people (the 'targets' of the advertisement) to make choices that are not strictly rational," researchers R.E. Ferner and D.K. Scott explained in a *Journal* report. "Rational prescribing should be based on logic, but advertisements do not depend on logical arguments for their most powerful effects: the advertisers may subvert us by appealing to our unconscious desires."

That marketing "strategy" isn't reserved just for patients. Medical doctors are targeted by drug advertising as well, and medical journals are filled with ads pushing one drug over another. The drug industry spends millions of dollars every year on advertising and, according to the report, "the money is well spent, since marketing undoubtedly influences the way that doctors prescribe."

One way of appealing to the emotions rather than the intellect is through the use of "symbols," the authors pointed out.

For example, a full-page, four-color ad appearing in the *American Medical News* was dominated by a huge, red, dew-sprinkled apple — the symbol of health. Under the photo of the apple were the words "Once-a-day... Rocephin." The intended emotional response was unmistakable: a Rocephin a day is as healthy as an apple a day. The **FACTS** were printed in tiny letters on the adjacent page: warnings, contraindications, precautions, adverse reactions (including pain, rash, diarrhea, headaches, dizziness, palpitations, and numerous other side effects).

"We should be on our guard," Ferner and Scott warned. "Advertisers use symbols in a way that implies a careful analysis of doctors' subconscious motives and aspirations. Doctors may themselves be reluctant to acknowledge these hidden feelings, but this reluctance makes them vulnerable."

Adding to the problem, according to a study in the *Annals of Internal Medicine,* is the fact that many of the ads for drugs that appear in medical journals are misleading. The researchers reviewed 109 ads appearing in 10 leading medical journals and found that 44% of them "would lead to improper prescribing if a doctor had no information about the drug other than that provided in the ad."

SOURCES:"Whatalotwegot — the messages in drug advertisements," by Ferner, R.E.; Scott, D.K. *British Medical Journal,* Dec. 24, 1994 v309 n6970 p1734(3).

"Drug advertisements misleading," by Luisa Dillner. *British Medical Journal,* June 13, 1992 v304 n6841 p1526(1).

Drug company admits physician kickbacks, fraud

When patients go to medical doctors, they know they'll probably walk out of the office with a prescription in hand or a recommendation for additional health care services.

What they don't know is how the doctor made the decision about which medicine to prescribe or service to recommend. Most people assume physician decisions are based on experience, knowledge and the best interest of the patient.

Unfortunately, that's not always the case. Too often, M.D.s make their decisions based on a brochure left by a drug company's sales rep. Or even, in some cases, on kickbacks received from the company.

In one case prosecuted by the federal government, Caremark International, an Illinois-based drug manufacturer, was accused of paying kickbacks to physicians to get them to recommend their services, which included growth hormones and the administration of intravenous drugs to homebound patients.

Although the company refused to admit any wrongdoing, it agreed to pay $161 million in civil and criminal fines — as well as an additional $42.3 million to resolve "good faith business disputes" — and did plead guilty to two counts of mail fraud.

SOURCE: "Caremark to pay $42.3 million to settle all remaining fraud charges," Associated Press release, *American Medical News,* April 8, 1996.

Drug companies spend billions on drug names to lure users

How much would you pay to have a company develop a clever marketing name for your product? $100? $500? $1,000?

For today's drug companies, the price for a name can reach as high as $150,000. "Branding," as the technique is called, is the creation of a memorable name which will help sell a drug, and there are a handful of top consulting companies specializing in developing "effective" names.

Find out more about health and chiropractic with these learning tools available through *The Chiropractic Journal*

Chiropractic First — Considered the best primer on chiropractic care available today, this book covers all aspects of chiropractic art, science and philosophy. Learn about the history of the profession, its view on health, how chiropractic can help you live a longer and more satisfying life and exactly what to expect when you set foot in a chiropractor's office. Paperback: $12.95

Under the Influence of Modern Medicine — The shocking truth about the failures of modern medicine. Everyone should read this book before swallowing another over-the-counter pill, visiting a medical doctor, or entering a hospital. The information here may save your life! Paperback: $12.95

Chiropractic: Compassion and Expectation — How much you benefit from chiropractic depends in large part on your understanding and expectations. This book gives you specific information about the scope, and limitations, of this fast-growing health care field. Paperback: $12.95

Health Watch Video — A fascinating talk-show program with Dr. Terry Rondberg and hosted by actress Maryann Sanders, providing important health information and step-by-step instructions on how to test yourself and loved ones for dangerous nerve interference. $29.95

Health Power Tapes — Four 40-minute audio tapes crammed with specific, practical information on how you and your family can optimize your health and well-being. Includes material on vaccines, children's health issues, aging and longevity, and much more! Narrated by Dr. Terry A. Rondberg. $39.95

Health Watch Newsletter — The highly respected newsletter which gives you the hidden facts about current medical research. These are the stories hidden from the American press. Every report is completely documented! 12 issues: $50.00

Use the order form below (photocopy acceptable) and save when you order two or more items.

❏ YES! I want to learn more about health and chiropractic. Please send the following items:

_____copies of **"Chiropractic First"** $ _____
_____copies of **"Under the Influence of Modern Medicine"** $ _____
_____copies of **"Chiropractic: Compassion and Expectation"** $ _____
_____copies of **"Health Watch Video"** $ _____
_____copies of **"Health Power Tapes"** $ _____
_____copies of **"Health Watch Newsletter"** $ _____

Subtotal $ _____
Tax (AZ res. 7.25%) $ _____
Postage & Handling $ _____
(Postage $3.25 for first item, $1.00 for each additional item)
TOTAL DUE $ _____

Name_____

Address_____

City/State/ZIP _____

Phone_____   FAX _____

❏ Check enclosed.   ❏ Bill my: ❏VISA ❏MasterCard ❏American Express

Account No. _____ Exp. Date _____

Signature of card holder _____

Make checks payable to and mail orders to: **The Chiropractic Journal,**
2950 N. Dobson Rd., #1, Chandler, AZ 85224 or fax credit orders to: 602-732-9313

or call 1-800-347-1011

Please allow 4–6 weeks for delivery. All sales are final — no refnds.